Eating Your Way to Health

—Dietotherapy in Traditional Chinese Medicine

by Cai Jingfeng

FOREIGN LANGUAGES PRESS   BEIJING

First Edition 1988
Second Edition 1996

ISBN 7-119-01885-X

© Foreign Languages Press, Beijing, 1996

Published by Foreign Languages Press
24 Baiwanzhuang Road, Beijing 100037, China

Printed by Beijing Foreign Languages Printing House
19 Chegongzhuang Xilu, Beijing 100044, China

Distributed by China International Book Trading Corporation
35 Chegongzhuang Xilu, Beijing 100044, China
P.O. Box 399, Beijing, China

Printed in the People's Republic of China

About the Author

Born in 1927, Cai Jingfeng graduated from the Hunan-Yale Medical College in 1954. He had served as resident physician at the Central People's Hospital, Beijing for over two years before he started to study systematically traditional Chinese medicine (TCM) for two and a half years. Since then he has been engaging in the research of Chinese medical history, including that of Chinese national minorities, for almost 40 years. He is a research fellow and professor at the China Academy of Traditional Chinese Medicine and is now specialized in medical history, Chinese and Tibetan. He has published over one hundred academic papers, including "The Origin and Evolution of the Theory of Channel-Collaterals," "On the Research of History of Ethnomedicine" and "Towards a Comprehensive Evaluation of Alternative Medicine." He has also published 20-some monographs, including *China's Tibetan Medicine, Medical Thangkas of the Four Medical Tantras (rGyud-bzRi)*. Professor Cai is the editor-in-chief or co-chief-editor of many TCM tool books, including *A Complete Dictionary of TCM*, and *WHO's WHO in Traditional Chinese Medicine*. He is also an advisory editor of the Beijing-based *Journal of TCM* (English edition) and Scotland-based international journal *Social Science & Medicine*. He is now the head of Section of History of Ethnomedicine, Chinese Medical Association.

CONTENTS

PREFACE

Since the publication of the first edition of *Eating Your Way to Health* in 1988, many readers have spoken highly of the book. Their comments encouraged me in my judgment that the Chinese technique of medical treatment through dietetic management, a unique science created by the Chinese over thousands of years, can be of great use. In recent years, more and more people from other countries are showing great interest in things Chinese, and Chinese dietotherapy has attracted special attention. Many foreign readers have expressed their wish for a more detailed and substantial introduction to Chinese dietotherapy. To meet such demands, the first edition has been revised and expanded to include some theoretical aspects of this science. This will provide a basis for the better understanding and mastery of dietotherapy's theoretical background and the use of its formulas. The number of examples of each medicinal diets has been increased to facilitate actual use. Clinical reports have been included along with some medicinal diets as testament to their efficacy. Experimental results reveal the scientific background underpinning the methodology.

I would like to express my heartfelt thanks to my assistant, Associate Professor Hong Wuli, who has helped me copy-edit and has typed out the entire text. Her wholehearted, unselfish devotion has proved essential to the completion of this work and to any accomplishment it may claim. I am also very grateful to Mr. Chen Yousheng of the Foreign Languages Press, who is an old friend of mine as well as the managing editor of this book. Without his encouragement, support and help, the publication of this book would have been totally impossible.

I sincerely hope that the present edition will be of still greater value to readers.

Cai Jingfeng

I. What Is Dietotherapy?

I suppose many readers are annoyed by taking medicines when they get ill. Some medicines are very peculiar, particularly those decoctions made from herbal compounds which are not only bitter, hot, sour and puckery, but also some of the tastes are so strange that one cannot even tell what they are! However, for the sake of treatment, what else can one do but pinch his nose and swallow it down.

Things might be even worse if your sick child is not obedient. He might run off as soon as he sees that medicine. What can you do then? You have to grab him, convince him to open his mouth, and then pour the medicine down his throat by pinching his nostrils. Unfortunately, if the process is not properly handled, liquid may escape down that trachea causing more complications, some even very serious. As for biomedicine, people are no more accustomed to its drugs than to the traditional ones. Though many of the bitter drugs are sugar-coated, children refuse to accept injections of any kind. Even worse, infants turn their backs toward the nurse and cry. Some even cry at their first glance of someone wearing a white uniform or gown.

How nice it would be if the decoction or bitter drugs to be taken could be made of foodstuffs or even taste like food!

Dietotherapy is a science which refers to the treatment of disease by the consumption of common foodstuffs; in China, these are sometimes called medicinal foods. The intake of food is necessary for the maintenance of everyone's daily life and activity. Food contains various nutrients which are essential to human life and provide the energy supply for the body's growth and activities. The old Chinese saying that "food is the first necessity for the people" reflects the vital importance of food in daily life.

Nutrients are essential for people during illness to overcome pathogenic factors and repair tissue damage, as well as to resist and prevent diseases while in good health.

3

The art of dietotherapy roughly includes the following: firstly, investigating the nature of food for preventing and treating diseases. In scurvy, a disease due to vitamin C deficiency, the eating of oranges, tangerines, or other fruit rich in vitamin C is helpful. Again, garlic behaves both as a food and as a remedy for bacillary dysentery. Secondly, investigating curative effects achieved by carefully selecting certain kinds of drugs and adding them to food to complement each other. For instance rice porridge is readily digested and nutritionally beneficial to patients. However, when radix discoreae, poria, or coix seeds are added, the porridge will have a strong anti-diarrhoea action through strengthening the spleen and improving digestion.

At present, the contents of dietotherapy are being greatly expanded. During the last few decades, cancer and cardiovascular diseases have replaced infectious diseases as the major enemy to human health. These two categories of disorders, especially cardiovascular diseases, are closely tied to food habits. Coronary heart disease, the most common cardiovascular disease, results from high blood cholesterol, which accumulates on the walls of the coronary vessels and leads to sclerosis. This process takes a long time to develop, perhaps eight to 10 years, or even as long as several decades. However, laboratory investigations reveal that signs of such pathologic changes in the coronary vessels can begin to appear during a person's 30s or even earlier. This reminds us that, so long as we pay attention to and reasonably adjust our daily food and drink, the process of arteriosclerosis can be greatly postponed or even prevented. Therefore, it is advisable, for macrobiotic purposes, to start one's healthy diet regime as early as possible to prevent the onset of obesity.

Dietotherapy should include two further closely interwoven aspects, namely, the development of cooking techniques to eliminate unpleasant tastes or odours from drugs, instead producing tasty and attractive foods, and the study of new foods with therapeutic potential and their recipes.

Moreover, dietotherapy also can be effective in the treatment of diseases such as AIDS, one of the current major threats to human life and health. Sufferings can be eased and the survival period greatly prolonged by dietotherapy. Chinese dietotherapy exerts extensive influence even in the Western world. There are many works on dietotherapy published in the Western languages, such as *Prince Wen Hui's Cook* by Bob Flaws of the United States, and *Chinese System of Food Cures, Prevention and Remedies* by Henry C. Lu of Canada.

Recently, the contents of traditional Chinese dietotherapy have been enriched by the further study of foods that are useful for preventing diseases and strengthening body resistance, cooking techniques for dietotherapeutic purposes, and the combining or contradiction of foodstuffs.

Chinese dietotherapy, as a natural therapy, has also been welcomed in many other countries. For instance, Mr. Sasada, a Japanese scholar, assessed in his paper entitled "Research into Modern Classics on Diet" those works relevant to foods from the period of the Song and Yuan dynasties onwards. In his opinion, ancient Chinese dietary study should embrace general works on food, and drink, delicacies of all sorts and also ordinary foods eaten by the common people. He concluded that such works amounted to as many as 38 in the Song-Yuan dynasties, 41 in the Ming Dynasty, and 40 in the Qing Dynasty.

The facts show that Chinese dietotherapy is a special branch of science with wide and unique contents.

II. A Time-Honoured Discipline, Historical Background

China, one of the world's most ancient civilizations, has a recorded history of several thousand years. Similar to the therapy with medicaments, Chinese dietotherapy also has a long history as well as copious contents, and has developed into a unique art of knowledge during its long course of evolution. And just as any branch of natural science, dietotherapy, as an independent discipline, has undergone the same process of maturity—from simplicity to complexity. Based on the analyses of literary materials and historical documents and archives, the history of dietotherapy can be divided into the following stages:

Primitive Stage (Remote Past, before the 21st Century B.C.):

An old Chinese proverb says that "Man has to rely on food for his livelihood." Of paramount importance for the primitive man was the acquisition of food so as to maintain life, growth, and reproduction. At that time, they had to rely solely on nature's beneficence. Food comes from nature and is multifarious. Under conditions of hunger, primitive man ate whatever he could obtain, regardless of its edibility. Among all the foods consumed, some might turn out to be uneatable or even poisonous. For instance, the achene Siberian cocklebur and rhubarb can cause serious bodily reactions, such as vomiting, diarrhoea, dizziness, etc. This might also include foods from animal kingdom. The chapter "Five Worms" from the *Book of Han Fei* by Han Fei (280 B.C.-233 B.C.) of the Warring States Period says: "In the remote antiquity, people ate fruits, gourds, clams, spoiled and notorious foods, which would cause damage to the stomach and intestines, resulting in various kinds of diseases." Similarly, the chapter "On the Cultivation of Morality" from the *Book of Prince Huai Nan* by Liu An (179 B.C.-122 B.C.) of the Western Han Dynasty says: "Ancient people ate plants, drank water, collected fruits from trees, and consumed animal flesh, from which diseases were apt to happen."

Obviously, ancient people were frequently disturbed and pained by diseases caused by inappropriate food and drink.

Through a long course of historical development, people learned how to tell those foods that were edible from those that were harmful. Master Huai Nan said, "Shen Nong tried everything, tasting the plants and sampling the waters in order to tell his people what to eat and what to avoid. Unfortunately, he himself was poisoned at least seventy times." This is a vivid example of how people barely escaped losing their lives due to poisonous materials in their never-ending search for food. Later, primitive man learned how to use fire; this enabled humans to eat cooked foods, which are not only more nutritious but also more tasty. As a result, people achieved stronger resistance to pathogenic bodily invasion. Cooked foods are, of course, a significant health asset. That is why *Li Wei, Han Wen Jia*, says: "Sui Ren (Flint Man) obtained fire by rubbing and drilling wood, and changed raw foods to cooked ones. Thus he instructed the people to prevent from suffering diseases." This illustrates the attempts at early prevention of disease caused by unsuitable foods.

All the above incidents happened unconsciously, with no thought given to any idea of dietotherapy or medicinal food. This is an important and difficult step forward towards the origin of dietotherapy.

Sprouting Stage (Xia-Spring and Autumn Period, the 21st century-476 B.C.):

In traditional Chinese medicine (TCM), there is an old saying that "medicaments and food share the same origin." Actually, food has an even closer and earlier relationship with human beings than medicines.

During this period, people found that appropriate diet had a direct bearing on the prevention and treatment of disease in human life; this idea was gradually shaped during the course of gradual improvement in cooking techniques. Interestingly, in Tibetan medicine, it is claimed that the earliest recognized disorder was dyspepsia, and the earliest medication, boiling water; this could be viewed as the earliest use of dietotherapy. However, in TCM, the record of soup (or decoction) solution is evidence of early dietotherapy prepared by Yi Yin, the chef of King Tang of the Shang Dynasty (c 16th-11th century B.C.). He was the person in charge of the imperial kitchen and was later promoted to the position of prime minister due to his contributions. Records show that Yi Yin used to discuss cooking with the king when they were talking about court affairs. *Lü Shi Chun Qiu, Ben Wei* (*Original Taste of Spring and Autumn of Master Lü*) mentions "the ginger from Yangpu, and the cinnamon from Zhaoyao." Both are warm and pungent food in nature and capable of resisting wind and cold pathogens. However, they are also flavouring materials for cooking. Obviously, preparations from these materials can be served both as edible soup and a medicinal decoction as well. This is the embryonic form of a medicinal diet. Though there are still controversies regarding the invention of decoctions, there is no doubt that the primitive form of dietotherapy appeared in the early Shang Dynasty (c 16th-11th century B.C.).

In fact, in the remains of Longshan Culture of the late Neolithic Period prior to the Shang Dynasty, there are liquid vessels of a type of pottery. Agriculture developed steadily during the Shang Dynasty. The inscriptions on tortoise shells and bones represent cereal plants, including crops, and millet. Moreover, literature also mentions "fragrant wine" (*chang*). So, it is doubtless that people produced wine on a large scale in this period. Wine is a type of drink with distinct simultaneous therapeutic effects that can be prepared as a medicinal drink. Since it has a higher potency of dissolving more materials than common water, it was extensively used for clinical purposes, including anesthetic application.

The art of diet had been highly developed during the Zhou Dynasty, when a rather complete system for diet and, in fact, an official post in charge of royal regulation on diet and food were established. In *Zhou Li Tian Guan* (*Celestial Official, Rituals of Zhou Dynasty*), there are four kinds of medical branches mentioned: dietary medicine, internal medicine, external medicine, and veterinary medicine. As indicated there, the responsibilities of dietary medicine include "governing of the king's food, drink, flavours, rare foods, etc." It can be seen that there is a close relationship between diet and health. By the end of the Spring and Autumn Period, the celebrated ancient philosopher, Confucius, mentioned the demands for dietary hygiene in *Lun Yu Xiang Dang* by saying, "Diet should be refined, cooking should be careful. Spoiled meat and fish with ghastly colour should be forbidden." Moreover, in another classic, *Shan Hai Jing* (*The Book of Mountains and Seas*), it is said that a kind of three-leg tortoise, when eaten, cures dropsy, while a kind of "Zhen" fish prevents the body from contracting diseases. All these demonstrated that a tremendous step had been made in dietotherapy during this period as compared with the past. It is obvious that the aim of a health-care diet was a definite and conscious behaviour of the people at this period.

Laying-Foundation Period (*Warring States Period-Han Dynasty*, 475 B.C.-220):

Through the accumulation of long-term experiences, it became apparent that the time was ripe to summarize the experiences and establish theories on dietotherapy. These were embodied in the relevant passages of the earliest medical classic, *Huang Di Nei Jing* (*Huangdi's Internal Classic*), which established the theoretical basis, not only for medicine as a whole, but also for dietotherapy, and still exerts profound influences on the practice of dietotherapy, as well as medicinal food.

In *Ling Shu* (*Miraculous Pivot*), it is mentioned the significance of food to human health, saying that "after food enters the stomach, its essence is absorbed to nourish all the viscera by passing through the passages for blood and *qi*." This demonstrates that food and drink are essential to the human body and its physiological functions. *Huangdi's Internal Classic* stresses that under all conditions, one should pay attention to diet for tackling diseases, even though medicines are pursued. One should not forget the importance of dietary nutrition for health.

Furthermore, it is emphasized in *Su Wen* (*Plain Questions*) that when dealing with disorders with "poisons" (referring to medicaments in this context), "cure the disease to 60 percent by drastic poisons, to 70 percent by average poisons, to 80 percent by light poisons, and to 90 percent by non-poisons. For the remaining illness not yet subdued, diets, including grains, meats, fruits and vegetables, are recommended. Do not violate these regulations, or the body health will be jeopardized." One can see that priority is given to diet instead of relying entirely on medicaments. Diet is even more reliable than non-poisonous drugs. In the classic, it is stated that, "to nourish the essence and spirit of the body, all kinds of grains, fruit, animals, and vegetables are needed." It means that as early as 2,500 years ago, ancient Chinese already advocated overall nutrition for a healthy body.

Since the ancient Chinese used to treat foods as medicaments, the theory for pharmacology is naturally also applicable for food and drink as well. It is claimed that foods also possess the attributions of four natures, cold, hot, warm, and cool; and five tastes, sweet, bitter, salty, sour and pungent. In applying dietotherapy, it is advisable to use foods antagonistic or allopathic in nature to the ailments; i.e., hot and warm food for cold diseases and vice versa. Among the five flavours: "Pungent and sweet yield the attribute of dispersal and belong to the *yang* principle. Sour and bitter yield the attribute of catharsis and belong to the *yin* principle. Salty also yields the attribute of catharsis and belongs to *yin*, while flat or neutral taste also yield the attribute of catharsis and belongs to *yang*." Thus foods are also categorized as *yin* and *yang* and should be carefully chosen when dealing with the treatment of ailments. It is obvious that the guiding principle of taste and nature of Chinese materia medica is crucial when applying dietotherapy.

Since there are different properties and flavours of diet, when consumed by the body, they yield biased action. It is stated in the same classic that "When the foods with different flavours are taken by the body, each flavour goes to what it prefers. The sour goes to the liver; the bitter, to the lungs; the sweet, to the spleen; the pungent, to the lungs; and the salty, to the kidneys." The work denotes the affinity of a diet to the visceral organs. In utilizing dietotherapy, these must be taken into consideration. Moreover, the classic also claims that "the liver used to suffer acuteness which should be eased by sweet food, the heart used to suffer leisure which should be treated by sour food; the spleen used to suffer dampness which should be checked by bitter food; the lung used to suffer adverse gas flowing which should be checked by bitter food, too; the kidney used to suffer dryness, which should be corrected by pungent food." Furthermore, "since the liver favours dispersion, it needs pungent food to disperse. Therefore, pungent benefits the liver while sour reduces it. Since the heart favours soft, it needs salty food to soften. Therefore, the salty benefits the heart while sweet reduces it. Since the spleen favours leisure, it needs sweet food to relax. Therefore, bitter reduces the spleen and sweet benefits it. Since the lungs favour preservation, it needs sour food to preserve. Therefore, the sour benefits the lungs, and pungent reduces them. Since the kidneys favour hardness, they need bitter food to harden. Therefore, the bitter benefits the kidneys and salty reduces them." All these theoretical ideas serve as guiding principles in dietotherapeutic practice.

Based on these ideas, people classified various foods into groups for indications and contraindications during clinical application. In the *Su Wen*

(*Plain Questions*), it is claimed that, "Since liver gives rise to green colour, sweet food, including rice, beef, dates, sunflower, is indicated. Since the heart gives rise to red colour, sour food, including beans, dog meat, plums, and chives, is indicated. Since the lungs give rise to white colour, bitter food, including wheat, mutton, apricots, Chinese onion bulb, is indicated. Since the spleen gives rise to yellow colour, salty food, including soybeans, pork, chestnuts, giant hyssop, is indicated. Since the kidneys give rise to black colour, pungent food, including millet, chicken, peaches, scallions, is indicated." Contraindicated foods are also mentioned here. This is a demonstration of dietotherapy based on a variety of visceral manifestations in illness. The only 12 recipes preserved in *Huangdi's Internal Classic* reveal a dietotherapy flavour. Among them, eight recipes contain such food as rice, cinnamon, wine, pork fat, horse fat, glutinous rice, sparrow's egg, abalone and Chinese prickly ash, as ingredients and the recipes are prepared in the forms of decoctions, pills, wine or paste. The indications for such recipes include diseases from internal medicine, gynecology, and surgery. This definitely shows that by then, dietotherapy was being extensively applied clinically.

The popularization of dietotherapy is further evidenced by the famous physician Zhang Zhongjiang's works in the Han Dynasty (206 B.C.-220): *Shang Han Lun* (*Treatise on Febrile Disease*) and *Jin Kui Yao Lüe* (*Synopsis of Prescriptions from Golden Chamber*). Taking the decoction of cinnamon-twig in *Treatise on Febrile Disease* for instance. Among the five ingredients it contains, four, including cinnamon twig, Chinese dates, rice and ginger, are all foods in common use. The decoction is to be taken with hot rice-porridge. Obviously, this is a typical dietary recipe. Other medicinal foods in the text include bee honey and rice. Moreover, food contraindication is another main dietary principle in this period. *Huangdi's Internal Classic* mentions in *Plain Questions* that, "Five flavours, when taken into the body, have their own preference. Since sourness prefers tendon, extra consumption of the sour would cause anuria. Since salt prefers blood, extra consumption of salty food would cause thirst. Since the pungent prefers *qi*, extra consumption of pungent diets would cause heartburn. Since the bitter prefers bone, extra consumption of bitter would cause vomiting. And since the sweet diet prefers muscles, extra consumption of sweet food would cause heartache." In another chapter of the same book, it is stated that over-consumption of various flavours also causes disorders, including obstruction of vessels with colour changes due to too much salty food, dropping of hair and withering of skin due to too much bitter food, spasm of tendons and dry nails due to too much pungent food, wrinkles and calluses in the muscles with turning down of lips due to too much sour food, and pain in the bone and dropping of hair due to too much sweet food. Though the above descriptions somewhat mechanically stick to the theory of Five-Phase Evolution, yet, in principle, the relation between improper food and disease incidence is convincing. Moreover, Zhang Zhongjing also mentioned contraindications among antagonistic foods by claiming that some foods are in mutually conflict and should not be taken at the same time, or, indeed, should be mutually avoided.

Historical records reveal that some dietotherapy monographs were written during this period. According to *Han Shu Yi Wen Zhi* (*Catalogue in Book of the Han Dynasty*) and others, these include *Shen Nong* and *Huangdi's Dietetic Contraindications, Dietetic Recipes, Canon of Food, Taiguan's Canon of Diet*, etc.

The stage of laying a foundation exerts a profound influence on the development of dietetics in later generations.

Stage of Formation (*Three Kingdoms Period-Tang Dynasty 220-907*):

On the basis of the previous period of theoretical foundation, further accumulation of experience has resulted in the integration of practice under the guidance of theory and eventually has led to the formation of an independent discipline, Chinese dietotherapy, in this period.

During the Eastern Jin Dynasty (317-420), though Ge Hong, a celebrated physician, did not devote any special chapters in his work to dietotherapy, he applied a lot of dietotherapeutic methods. Because the treating principle of convenience, simplicity and effectiveness he advocated is in line with the basic idea of dietotherapy. In his *Zhou Hou Bei Ji Fang* (*Handbook of Prescriptions for Emergency*), he mentioned beriberi, the earliest record in Chinese medical history, and advised the application of processed beans infused in wine for three days for its treatment. The remedy is also good for prevention. Other dietetic recipes include fresh juice from pears for coughing, honey water and baked tortoiseshell powder for promoting lactation, potato with white chicken juice plus black male duck juice for edema, and bean rice or bean juice for beriberi.

In the Southern-Northern Dynasties (420-581), Tao Hongjing, in his *Ben Cao Jing Ji Zhu* (*Variorum of Classic of Herbology*), the second milestone in the history of Chinese pharmacology, collected a large amount of medicinal foods, including crab, fish, pork, wheat, Chinese dates, bean, kelp, scallion, ginger, balsam pear, totalling some one hundred kinds. It also mentions food hygiene, saying, "Tortoise with protruding eyes should be forbidden," and "A fish with red eyes is not suitable for making soup." Also mentioned were mutually conflicting foods like mutton and cock, sheep's liver and plum with prickly ash, etc.

It was not until the Sui and Tang dynasties (581-907) that dietotherapy became an independent discipline. In his *Bei Ji Qian Jin Fang* (*Valuable Prescriptions for Emergency*), Sun Simiao, the "medical king" in the Chinese medical history, devoted a separate chapter to dietotherapy, indicating that the discipline had come into being. The chapter is divided into five sections. The first section, devoted to theory, says: "He who doesn't know dietotherapy is unable to cure diseases. Only those applying diet for treatment are superb physicians." It indicates that a physician's qualifications were appraised for his use of dietotherapy. This work also stresses: "As a physician, one must first probe its etiology to search out what is wrong. Then, dietotherapy is recommended first, with drugs to follow, provided dietotherapy is applied to no avail." Hence, dietotherapy was apparently the first choice for treatment in that period.

Then he mentioned 164 kinds of medicinal foods, including 29 kinds of fruits, 58 vegetables, 27 grains and 40 animals, each with a detailed description of its nature, flavour, actions, channel-tropism, indications and contraindications and methods of administration.

Next came a pharmacological book specializing in dietotherapy, *Shi Wu Ben Cao* (*Dietetic Herbology*), written by Meng Xian (621-713), a native of Ruzhou or Liangxian County (now Linru, Henan Province). Unfortunately, this monograph was lost long ago; only some of its texts were quoted by other relevant herbal works, such as *Ben Cao Shi Yi* (*Supplement of Herbology*) by Chen Cangqi of the Tang Dynasty (618-907), *Isimbo* by Damba Mototane of Japan, *Da Guan Ben Cao* (*Herbology of Daguan Period*) and *Zheng He Ben Cao* (*Herbology of Zhenghe Period*) of the Song Dynasty (960-1279). A recovered edition was compiled and published by utilizing the quoted texts from these books. Altogether, there are 227 kinds of medicinal foods presented in three volumes. For each food, the source, indications, flavour and nature and processing methods are given. For instance, under coriander, we find 11 recipes for the treatment of poisoning from meat, bleeding, body odour, dental caris, visceral deficiency, headache, skin rash, pox and children's baldish ulcers. One of the recipes points out that "together with raw vegetable, coriander cures diarrhoea. When wrapped with cake and eaten, the result is even better." Another example is Chinese yam. "It can be made as steamed bread with flour. Mixed with honey or prepared as soup, or powder, all good for medical use. When dried for use, the result will be even more satisfactory." It is obvious that a medicinal diet was used for treating diseases and keeping fit. It was also emphasized that one should pay attention to regional difference when applying dietotherapy, since results may depend on different places.

Actually, in the Tang Dynasty, medicinal food was rather common. Sun Simiao applied mutton soup with Radix Astragali seu Hedysari as a blood tonic. This recipe became quite popular among people as a common nourishing recipe. In another medical work of the same period, the *Wai Tai Mi Yao* (*Medical Secret of an Official*) carries some 6,000 recipies, among them medicinal diets were also common. An apriconut decoction, containing apricot nut, Chinese prickly ash, honey, sugar, ginger juice, pork kidney, was to be prepared as a cake with dry ginger and flour. Moreover, ginger juice with honey for cold dysentery and bean juice for sudden bleeding are all typical medicinal foods. This book also provides contraindications of foods used against diseases, including the avoidance of cold and raw food, greasy food and wine.

In addition to *Dietetic Herbology*, there are also other dietotherapeutic monographs, of which *Shi Yi Xin Jian* (*Mirror of Dietotherapy*) is worthy of mentioning. Though it was lost in early times, some of its remaining contents were quoted in the Korean masterpiece, *Yi Fang Lei Ju* (*Classified Recipes*), in which both theoretical and practical contents were all included, together with 200 dietotherapeutic recipes.

In summary, dietotherapy was greatly developed and an independent discipline was thus formed, laying a firm foundation for the further development of the discipline in the next stage.

Overall Development Stage (*Song-Qing Dynasties, 960-1911*):

On the basis of the previous period when an independent discipline of dietetic therapy had been formed, the Northern Song Dynasty saw a relative stable society and environment. It is particularly interesting that some of its emperors were personally interested in medicine and substantially involved in medical activities; therefore, effective measures were adopted to promote its development. A few prominent examples: The Bureau of Collating Medical Books was established for the collating, checking and systematizing of ancient medical works; another institution, called the Taiping Bureau of Drug Compounding for Benevolence, was also founded. These greatly promoted the development of the traditional Chinese medicine in this period, and the discipline of dietotherapy as well. Thus this period saw a stage of overall development.

Through investigation of the three voluminous works on recipes of the Song Dynasty, it is obvious that a considerable part of their contents is devoted to dietotherapy. In both *Taiping Shenghui Fang* (*Taiping's Recipes for Holy Benevolence*) and *Shenji Zonglu* (*A Comprehensive Record of Holy Benevolence*), special chapters are devoted to dietotherapy. In the former, chapters 96 and 97 of the 100-chapter book are related to dietotherapy in which 160 recipes are recorded, amounting to 1 percent of the total. Altogether, 28 kinds of disorders are dealt with there, including stroke, wind pathogens, consumption, diabetes, diarrhoea, vomiting, deafness, gonorrhoea, hemorrhoids, deficient spleen and stomach, and all sorts of dysentery. It should be pointed out that among these recipes, medicinal food occupies a rather high proportion, appearing in the form of drinks, soups, cakes, and particularly gruels, including those made of processed beans, peach, kernels, apricot kernels, black beans, and carp and gruel of Job's tear. This demonstrates clearly that gruel represented a large proportion of medicinal foods during this period. In Zhang Zhongjiang's *Shang Han Lun* (*Treatise on Febrile Disease*), gruel is applied as an adjuvant therapy for strengthening the action of decoction. As time goes by, this form of dietotherapy by gruel has become the mainstream of traditional Chinese medicine (TCM), specifically, never seen in other contemporary medical systems. During this period, medicinal diets further developed in multiple form, including medicinal wines, soups, cakes, noodles, powders, etc.

The Yuan Dynasty (1271-1368) saw the first monograph on TCM

nutriology, *Yin Shan Zheng Yao* (*Orthodox Essentials of Diet*), written by the Mongolian medical official, Hu Sihui, with far wider coverage than any of his predecessors. This monograph extends its scope from former dietotherapy ideas to more modern nutritional notions by stressing the hygiene of food and drink and the prevention of disease on a nutritional background. This author emphasized: "Those who are conversant with macrobiotics used to eat before hunger, without too much food, and to drink before thirst, again without too much beverage." In this three-volume monograph, the best foods are suggested as nourishing agents for normal people to strengthen their bodies. It mentions only common foods such as mutton and sheep's organs, instead of those rare and "precious" foods of dainties and delicacies. The author was the first to expound foods from a nutritional background in the history of TCM. In the first chapter, for instance, he mentioned the preparation and cooking of many daily foods, including 16 kinds of soup, 6 types of powder, 8 kinds of flour, 4 kinds of syrup and 4 kinds of gruel, as well as the making of other foods, such as steamed bread, dumplings, jams, cakes and stuffed steamed breads.

In the same book, many dietotherapy menus and recipes for various diseases are also listed. Following are common examples: for vomiting and gastric hypofunctions, 4 *liang* (1 *liang* = 1.7637 ounces) of flour, plus 3 *qian* (1 *qian* = 5 grams) of peel from prickly ash pepper tree; for cold epigastric pain, 1/2 *liang* of powdered lasser galangal in rice, or 2 *ge* (1 *ge* = 198.1 ml) of juice from rehmannia root, cooked in rice porridge; for coughing with stuffy chest and asthma, porridge with 3 *liang* of peeled peach kernels with tips discarded, and porridge of Herba Malva for anuresis; for deficient kidney and emaciation, a black ox-marrow soup made of 1/2 *jin* (1 *jin* = 0.5 kilogramme) of marrow from a black ox, 1/2 *jin* of rehmmania juice, plus 1/2 of *jin* honey; for soreness and pain in leg and waist: 4 hoofs from a deer plus 2 *qian* of old tangerine peel and 2 *qian* of tsaoguo root. These are all typical of medicinal diets. In its last chapter, 203 kinds of diets are classified under seven categories, i.e., cereals, beasts, birds, fish, fruits, vegetables and processed products. All tastes and effects are expounded. The advent of this monograph marked the high level and maturation of the science of dietotherapy which bears two major characteristics: On the one hand, it mainly reflects the dietetic habits of northern China because the author is from that area; on the other, it features the customs and habits of national minorities, the Mongolian and Uygur people among others. Since the ruling class was the monarchy of the Mongolian people, many special Mongolian specialties are included to meet their needs, including fruits like Bazan kernel and Bisda, and spicy flavours like Masdaji, saffron, Suolotuoyin, Hasini, Huihui green, etc.

Other works include Wu Rui's *Ri Yong Ben Cao* (*Daily Herbology*), Luo Juzhong's *Shi Zhi Tong Shuo* (*General Discourse for Dietotherapy*), and Zheng Qiao's *Shi Jian* (*Mirror for Foods*), which reflect the development of dietotherapy from various approaches. For instance, Luo Juzhong held that dietotherapy is "one of the measures for preventing disease by superb physicians," stressing the importance of diets.

The Ming and Qing dynasties marked the stage of comprehensive development in dietotherapy. Nearly all works in herbology give considerable space to dietotherapy, demonstrating the close relationship between the two sciences. The renowned Li Shizhen's *Ben Cao Gang Mu* (*Materia Medica*), a pharamacopoeia in 52 volumes, is an example; in addition to discussing hundreds of edible foods, it contains many recipes of dietotherapy. In volumes 3 and 4, under the category "Major Drugs for Treatment," the work offers several hundred recipes for over 100 kinds of diseases. These include black chicken boiled with wine for a type of deficient wind disorder; soybean products and red beans, bean curd and fennel prepared with pork fat as pills for exhaustion; various kinds of porridge for spleen-stomach illness; mutton with raw garlic for cold dysentery; chicken with hen's eggs for dysenteric abdominal pain, etc.

There are also herbal monographs revolving around the same subject. In Zhu Shu's *Jiu Huang Ben Cao* (*Herbology for Famine*), a total of 414 kinds of wild plants are recorded as cultivated in the garden, with their roots, stems, barks, leaves, flowers and fruits portrayed; also, the original places of production, titles, nature and cooking methods are mentioned. Although these plants are not for daily use, yet they still are of practical significance during famine disasters. It demonstrates that even by then, dietotherapeutic nutriology had developed to a new level.

The compounding of dietotherapy recipes also revealed a new development in this period. In Chapter 98 of Xu Chunpu's *Gu Jin Yi Tong* (*Medical*

Keylinks of Ancient and Contemporary Periods), a great variety of preparations for dietetic nutriology are recorded. These include tea, liquids, soups, vinegars, soybean sauces, vegetables, animal flesh, fresh fruits, butter, curd, cheese, and honey preserved fruits, most of which are nutritious.

Special attention was paid to dietetic therapy for the elderly, as well as patients suffering various sorts of diseases during the Ming and Qing dynasties. Among the many monographs, Gao Lian's *Zun Sheng Ba Qian* (*Eight Chapters for Longevity*) mentions in full detail many foods and beverages for the elderly. It also includes 38 kinds of porridge and 32 types of soup. Cao Cishan's *Lao Lao Heng Yan* (*Maxim for Respecting the Elderly*) of the Qing Dynasty gives a detailed list of various porridge suitable for the elderly, saying, "Porridge is beneficial to health, especially for the elderly." The work divides various kinds of porridge into three categories: superior class, "light in nature and tasty"; intermediate class, "a little bit inferior to the superior ones"; inferior class, "heavy and turbid in nature." It also holds that "for the elderly, porridge can be provided all the day. Whenever one feels hungry, porridge can be taken. It not only strengthens your health, but also prolongs your life remarkably." Altogether, 36 kinds of porridge are included under the superior category, 27 under the intermediate, and 37 under the inferior one. Among other items, porridges contain lotus seeds, cogon fruit, lotus roots, apricot kernels, walnuts, chrysanthemum and peppermint. Leaves of Chinese wolfberry are superior, those with poria, red beans, dates, longan and milk, intermediate; and those containing Radix Rehmania, Chinese onion white, sheep's liver and carp, vulgar. All of these are medicinal gruels for strengthening body health, and to be administered as a tonic for the infirm, especially the elderly.

Monographs on dietotherapy are abundant in this period. In addition to those above, at least over 30 works in this field were produced, mainly on herbology. The famous ones include Shen Lilong's *Shi Wu Ben Cao Hui Chuan* (*A Collection of Dietetic Herbology*), Lu He's *Shi Wu Ben Cao* (*Herbologic Foods*), Ning Yuan's *Shi Jian Ben Cao* (*Mirror of Dietetic Herbology*), Li Shizhen's *Shi Wu Ben Cao* (*Dietetic Herbology*), Wu Wenbing's *Shi Yi Ben Cao* (*Herbology for Dietetic Herbology*), and Fei Boxing's *Shi Jian Ben Cao* (*Mirror of Dietetic Herbology*). Other works dealing with the preparation, cooking and adjustment of foods and beverages, as well as dietotherapeutic recipes and nutriology, include Jia Ming's *Yin Shi Xu Zhi* (*Guides for Foods and Drinks*), Song Gongyu's *Yin Shi Shu* (*Book of Foods and Drinks*), Yuan Mei's *Sui Yuan Shi Dan* (*Sui Yuan's Recipes*), Zhang Mu's *Tiao Ji Yin Shi Bian* (*Differentiation of Foods and Drinks for the Sick*) and Wang Mengying's *Suixiju Yin Shi Pu* (*Suixiju's Recipes*), some of which are still of practical importance even today. These are part of the valuable heritage of Chinese medicine.

The idea of advocating vegetarian food was further developed and highly stressed in this period. As early as in *Huangdi's Internal Classic*, addiction to certain foods were warned against, especially greasy foods: "Too many greasy foods are vulnerable to boils and carbuncles." Unfortunately, for a long period, though greasy foods were criticized, this idea was not upgraded to a dietotherapeutic standpoint. In *Yin Shan Zheng Yao* (*Orthodox Essentials of Diet*), many nutritious foods are listed. However, most of them are greasy and fatty foods from animals (which might be due to the author's home in northern China). Northerners and Mongolians are accustomed to animal foods. As time passed, the problem of fatty foods harmful to health aroused the attention of the medical field. For instance, Lu He's *Shi Wu Ben Cao* (*Dietetic Herbology*) advocates that more millet should be planted, indicating that crops and vegetables are more beneficial and helpful to bowel movements. It held that "the five cereals are nourishing foods bestowed by nature." "All vegetables are grown from the earth, which belongs to *yin* and nourishes the *yin* principle of the body," it said, "while *shu* (vegetables) are good for *shutong* (catharsis)."

In short, Chinese dietotherapy has a long history with rich knowledge. It will continue to contribute to the health of the Chinese, as well as other people worldwide, provided it can be explored by modern scientific measures.

III. Features of Dietotherapy

Just like any other branch of clinical science in the traditional Chinese medicine (TCM), dietotherapy has been used to apply its own theoretical points as guidelines through its long process of practice. This eventually formed the special features of today's dietotherapy, including TCM theory as its core, the emphasis of treatment based on overall analysis of disease manifestations, common origin of food and medicine, and the unity of nature and flavour between food and medicine. It also emphasizes food indications and contraindications, protection of the functions of spleen and stomach, and promotion of absorption and assimilation of medicinal food to its greatest extent. In other words, the theory of dietotherapy is closely related to that of the TCM, and developed side by side with the latter. It plays a very important role in the prevention, treatment and health care of the Chinese people. In a certain sense, Chinese dietotherapy is even more effective in practice than modern nutriology.

A. The Common Origin of Medicine and Food

There is an old saying: "Traditional medicine and food share a common origin." In other words, medicine and food have the same origin, but different usages. In remote prehistoric times, there must have been a period when medicine and food were both eaten indiscriminately without any distinct demarcation. This is simply due to the fact that primitive people could not yet tell medicine from food. When they were badly in need of food, and they, extremely hungry, might eat anything, which could result in a marked reaction to the body such as vomiting, diarrhoea or vertigo. It was not until a long time later that people began to differentiate a few substances which contained clear therapeutic action from common foods.

Legend has it that around the 11th century B.C., King Tang of the Shang Dynasty had an excellent chef named Yi Yin, who also cooked soups for his king when he was ill. Having eaten a few bowls of soup, the king would then recover. Hence Yi Yin is reputed to be the inventor of decoctions. Whatever the real story, this legend suggests that soups and decoctions share a common origin. This common origin of food and medicine is also reflected in the case of wine. Wine has been very popular since ancient times. However, it also became of great importance in medicine, so much that both the Chinese characters for "medicine" (醫) and "wine" (酒) share the same component " 酉 " as their radicals.

Then dietotherapy is based on this common origin of medicine and food. In traditional Chinese medicine, many common foods serve as medicines and many specific medicines are also commonly used foodstuffs. Among others, Chinese dates, ginger, cinnamon, Chinese prickly ash, Chinese onion, garlic, Chinese yam, liquor, vinegar, eggs, sesame, mung bean, apricot kernels and rice are the most common.

In brief, many natural products possess such a duality, and it is often difficult to say whether they are foodstuffs or medicine. Generally, we use the term "foodstuffs" for those edibles which are taken daily or quite often and can be consumed over a long period of time without detrimental effects; whereas those which are not palatable, nor in daily use and produce a distinct physiological reaction are called medicines or drugs.

Moreover, it is customary to get medicines from a drugstore or dispensary and foodstuffs from a grocery. It is interesting to note that in Western countries, some patented medicines are sold in the grocery. This phenomenon is actually the result of social progress and the division of work. As bestowed by nature, medicines are easy to distinguish from foods, and strictly speaking, most medicines are isolated from foodstuffs. A certain substance which revealed a marked reaction when swallowed and could not be taken repeatedly was isolated from ordinary foodstuffs and treated as "medicine." When the body is discomforted to such an extent that it becomes necessary to apply such "food" capable of producing dramatic action to cure that discomfort, this is treatment by use of "medicine." Gradually, medicines were isolated from the family of food. However, foodstuffs, such as cinnammon, Chinese dates, peppers, Chinese prickly ash, lotus roots, pumpkin seeds, walnuts, longan, crystal sugar, hawthorns, seeds of Job's tears and many other herbs, spices and natural products, can be bought from a herbalist or a grocery shop and are used both for daily cooking and as medicine.

In order to maintain normal daily activity, the body needs energy, which is supplied by food and drink. When the body requires energy, discomfort or abnormal sensations are felt. For instance, when one feels hungry and if food is not supplied in time, one may experience dizziness, palpitations, perspiration, and weakness. This is a temporary physiological reaction called hypoglycemia, and it can be immediately set right if food is supplied in time. Probably everyone has experienced this sensation at some time or another. However, this condition is not generally viewed as pathological, since it is a kind of physiological reaction. It can thus be seen that the two states are relative rather than absolute, with no sharp demarcation, just as in the case of food and medicine. Without food, the normal physiological state will change into a pathological one. This is evident when starvation occurred during wartime. A radically improper food supply, especially for those with special needs such as the elderly and pregnant women, would result in a breakdown of physical health.

These two concepts, the relative relationship between the pathological and normal condition and the common origin of food and medicine, provide the foundation and starting point for dietotherapy in traditional Chinese medicine.

B. The Nature and Flavour of Food

Traditional Chinese medicine lays great stress on the nature and flavour of materia medica, which have four characteristics: cold, hot, warm, and cool; and five flavours, salty, sour, sweet, bitter and pungent. In traditional Chinese medicine, the application of antagonistic or allopathic therapy is emphasized by using medicine with the opposite nature and flavour to that of the illness. Therefore, it is of great significance to explore and master the characteristics of medicines in order to achieve "neutralization," i.e., a harmonized state of the body.

Traditional Chinese medicine holds that the human body is healthy when it is in a harmonious state. A preponderance of any condition would result in disease. For instance, disease may manifest itself as cold or hot, deficient or excessive in nature. Acute diseases manifesting high fever, thirst, headache, deep-coloured urine, and yellow fur on the tongue surface, etc. are often said to be of a hot and excessive nature. Meanwhile, chronic diseases with a protracted duration, hypo-functions and bad circulation manifesting cold extremities, chills, emaciation, short breath, feeble pulse, bald tongue and debility, etc. are said to be cold and deficient in nature. For severe cases of hot diseases, cold remedies should be used; while for mild cases, cool remedies should be applied. In contrast, for those severe cold diseases, hot remedies are indicated; warm medicines are prescribed for mild diseases of a cold nature.

It goes without saying that since dietotherapy is a kind of treatment, it should obey the same principles as medicinal therapy in order to overcome the preponderance of any condition causing disorder. Since food and medicine are treated under the same principle, the property of foodstuffs is also differentiated into four categories: hot, warm, cold and cool for allopathic therapy when applying dietotherapy. In other words, similar attention should be paid to the nature and flavour of food and drink. For instance, among common foods, coriander is warm, pepper is hot, balsam pear is cold and bean curd is cool in nature. Moreover, baked, fried and broiled foods are all hot and dry in nature, while greasy and mucilaginous foods when eaten tend to transform themselves into heat or evil-hot and dampness. Vegetables and fruits, with few exceptions, are cool and sour. Naturally, one must pay attention to the nature of these foods so as to achieve good results with treatment and in daily diet for pursuit of health and longevity. An illness of a hot nature will be worsened by eating mutton, dog meat, chicken, pepper, cinnamon, dried ginger, longan or lichee—which are all of a warm or hot nature. Similarly, those suffering from diseases of a cold nature should avoid taking foods, such as sugar cane, water chestnut, watermelon, balsam pears, etc., which are believed cold or cool in nature.

Regarding the five flavours (salty, sour, sweet, bitter and pungent), each has its own pharmacological action, which has been determined by theory and through long experience and practice in daily life. Accordingly, traditional Chinese medical theory claims that salty medicines are good at softening lumps, and pungent medicines for dispersing the vital energy throughout the body; this is helpful to eliminate evil pathogens, and is commonly applied for the common cold and flu. TCM holds that sweet medicines are good for deficient diseases, although excess sweets are harmful to the appetite; sour medicines for astringent action, treating loss of body fluid, such as in diarrhoea or excess sweating, and for activating blood circulation; and bitter medicines for antipyretic use, elimination of dampness and stimulating the appetite.

Actions from the five flavours of foods are basically the same as those from medicines. Bitter foods are antipyretic, such as fermented soya beans, balsam pears, animal bile, etc.; sweet foods are fluid secretion promoting, *yin* nourishing and also antipyretic, such as lotus roots, potatoes, Radix Rehmaniae, Radix Dioscorea (Chinese yam), Radix Polygonati (sealwort), Semen *coicis* (coix seed), sweet potatoes, sugar cane and watermelons (most starch-rich foods are in this class). Sour foods are astrigent, blood activating and stagnation eliminating, such as hawthorns, wild jujubes, vinegar, apricots, tomato and the like. Pungent foods are capable of dispersing evil cold and wind, such as Chinese onion, ginger, prickly ash peel, mustard and chilli. These are commonly applied at the initial stage of the common cold, when the invading cold and wind still remain in the superficial part of the body. Salty food refers to innate salty foods rather than those processed with salt. For instance, foods from the sea such as seaweed and kelp are innately salty foods, and are capable of softening lumps, such as goiters, tubercular lymph glands, etc. Meanwhile, salty foods such as processed salty meat or fish do not possess such capacity.

In order to achieve satisfactory therapeutic results, it is essential to take the nature and flavour of foodstuffs into overall account. In medicinal therapy, drugs of a hot nature, like ephedra and cinnamon twigs, are applied in cases of severe cold diseases, while for mildly cold ailments, only honeysuckle flower and forsythia fruit would be applied. These rules are similarly applicable in dietotherapy, and the action of the food, whether mild or drastic, should be recognized. For instance, onions and ginger are strongly hot, while raw brown sugar and turnip are warm. They should be chosen for treatment according to the severity of the ailment. However, most foods always possess two or even more kinds of flavour. Some are both sour and sweet, others both pungent and bitter, while their nature may be rather simple, either hot or cold, warm or cool. Hence one must have a thorough understanding of their nature and flavour in order to use them effectively to cure diseases.

As a rule, severe and acute diseases should be treated by medicines or a combination of medicines with dietotherapy; for cronic ailments, dietotherapy is highly recommended. Medicines, no matter how simple their action, often

24

produce certain unexpected and disadvantageous side effects, some even harmful to the body. With dietotherapy, such shortcomings can be avoided even over a long period of therapy.

C. Characteristics of Medical Theory in Dietotherapy

Viewing the human body as a holistic organism with viscera and channels as its structural essence, TCM treats it as the unity of the two opponents, *yin* and *yang*. Traditional Chinese medicine holds that the occurrence and evolution of disease is the process of loss of harmony between *yin* and *yang*, essentially a conflict between the body and various pathogenic factors. Therefore, it is imperative that, when treating a disorder—even a localized one—that the physician should attend to the patient from an overall viewpoint instead of dealing it topically with either medicinal or dietetic therapies. Taking agalactosis or hypogalactosis as an example, one should not focus one's attention on secretion of the mammary gland; rather, the postpartum condition should be taken into account. In TCM, it is usually claimed that these conditions are due to the obstruction of the liver channel supplying the mammary gland; yet, the postpartal deficiencies of *qi* and blood of the mother should also be considered as the root cause. On this basis, nourishing and invigorating the patient's *qi* and blood, the provenance of milk secretion, should be given preferential consideration. Tonics for *qi* and blood, such as ginseng, Radix Astragali seu Hedysari and Si Wu (four-ingredient) decoction always effectively provide desired results.

The principle, "treatment based on differential diagnosis and an overall analysis of syndromes," is the basic feature of TCM. It is composed of two integral parts, i.e., differential diagnosis and overall analysis of syndromes, and treatment. The former does not represent the simple listing of all signs and symptoms; instead, it is the comprehensive analysis of all symptoms and signs. This is especially true for lingual fur and pulse manifestations on which the intrinsic connections are drawn so as to find the root causes, pathogenesis, locations of lesions and pathological changes for the formulation of therapeutic principles and concrete treating measures. The therapeutic approaches also include the so-called "treating different disorders with the same therapy," and "treating the same disorder with different therapeutic approaches." All these principles are also applicable to dietotherapy. Taking nephritis with edema as its main manifestation, for instance, this ailment is divided into *yin* and *yang* types, which essentially belong to deficient and excessive types, respectively. Therefore, the respective treatment should be to strengthen body resistance and its digestive functions, and to expel pathogens by antiphlogistics and diuretics, respectively. When treating the problem with dietotherapy, the same principle should be applied. For *yang* or excessive type, onion-white porridge, five-peel drink, porridge of Semen Pharbitidis and porridge of Radix Phyto-laccae are prescribed. As for the excessive type of damp-heat, red bean diets are indicated. For the deficient type with cold in the lower part of the body, a diet containing cinnamon, aconitum, black beans, and black sesame is essential; carp porridge or soup is also highly recommended (*Orthodox Essentials of Diet*). In treating edema, the idea of limiting salt intake came to TCM much earlier; this is recorded in Chapter 4 of the *Handbook of Prescriptions for Emergency*, which orders the avoidance of too much salt and water intake.

The principle of maintaining adjustment and harmony between dieto-therapy and medicinal therapy should be emphasized; hence, coordination between dietitian and physician is crucial for the treatment of diseases.

D. Herbological Theory Applicable for Selection of Foodstuffs

On the basis of an overall analysis of syndromes for differential diagnosis and treatment, the principle of a given dietotherapy is to be established, including the selection of food and medicine and its compounding. This is a crucial part of dietotherapy. Experience demonstrates that besides the flavour and nature of foods, the herbological theory of channel tropism and acting orientation are also of great significance. Herbologically, the problem of channel tropism is based on the theory of relations between the viscera and channel. This is the selective action of herbs on the organism and is of practical importance. In TCM, since the lesion of ailment used to transmit from one viscera to another and mutually the involved viscera are affected; hence when compounding a recipe, it is of practical necessity that all the involved channels should be taken into account. This theory is also applicable in dietotherapy. For instance, for habitual constipation in the elderly, the recipe in common use is Semen Pruni porridge, containing Semen Pruni, rice and bee honey. These are all sweet in flavour with respective channel tropism to the spleen, stomach and lungs. The results are always satisfactory. Another example is Fructus Mori porridge, made of Semen Mori, glutinous rice and crystal sugar. It is good for checking dizziness, vertigo, insomnia, and forgetfulness. This recipe is based on the channel tropism of Semen Pruni, and glutinous rice is good to liver and spleen, respectively. Obviously, channel tropism is also important in dietotherapy.

Acting orientation of floating, sinking, ascending and descending indicates the tendency and the action of a drug. Ascending and floating refer to a drug's tendency to behave upward and outward, with the capability to disperse and eliminate superficial pathogens, dissipate and eliminate cold-evil and emesis and ascend the *yang* principle; whereas, descending and sinking refer to those drugs which tend to behave downward and inward. These are also capable of pressing down the abnormal flow of *qi*, depressing the uprushing *yang* principle while decreasing sweating, catharlsis, and antiemesis. These theories are also applicable and important in dietotherapy, though not so important and universally applied as they are in pharmacology. However, for those "collapsed syndromes," such as rectal prolapse, gastroptosis and uterine prolapse, dietotherapy, plus drugs of floating and ascending nature (such as ginseng, Radix Astragali seu Hedysari, and Rhizoma Qimifugae) are always applied. Meantime, for diseases located in the lower part of the body (lower *jiao*), sinking and descending drugs are often applied, all with satisfactory results.

In administrating dietotherapy, all these theoretical problems should be taken into account in a flexible way, instead of being followed stereotypedly. Under the guidance of these principles, new dietotherapeutic recipes can be formulated.

E. Protection of Stomach Energy

In TCM, the spleen and stomach are treated as important visceral organs of digestion and temporary storage of foods. TCM holds that one of the physiological features of the spleen and stomach is the ascending and descending nature of their function, i.e., it differentiates the clear portion from the turbid and supplies the body with nutrients. In the treatment of diseases, TCM emphasizes the importance of stomach function, the so-called stomach-*qi*, the condition of which is closely related to the physiology of other viscera.

Hence, the strengthening of the stomach-*qi* to bring its function into full play so as to provide the body with plenty of nutrients and energy is the keylink for the success of dietotherapy; otherwise, the therapy will be doomed to failure. TCM accumulates rich experiences on how to protect and enhance stomach-*qi*. One must bear in mind stomach-*qi* whenever treating any kind of a disease. Advocation of dietary therapy is encouraged; dietotherapy is given priority in various sorts of disease treatment. If dietotherapy fails to be effective, drug therapy is then recommended. This is one of the general rules for therapy in ancient TCM.

It is essential, therefore, to take concrete and implicit steps to protect stomach-*qi*. These include the food intake behaviour adapted to the changes of four seasons, advocacy of well-cooked and soft diets, instead of raw, hard and cold foods, advocacy of frequent meals rather than one sudden and over-full meal plus other immoderate food and drink habits. It is not unusual in Chinese dietotherapy to add some remedies capable of promoting digestion, warming the body interior, regulating the flow of *qi*, as well as aromatic remedies which are good for the stomach, into the food during the cooking process. However, aromatic drugs, though beneficial to the promotion of digestive functions when given in appropriate amounts, are not suitable for people of deficient temperament vulnerable to deficient or asthenic fire disorders. For a regular diet, it is significant to have good and palatable taste, fragrant smell, beautiful colour and attractive appearance so as to whet one's appetite. Similarly, dietotherapy needs the same characteristics, but with a great variety of natural sources possessing an attractive appearance and smell. It should be well compounded so as to stimulate the appetite instead of being simplified and repeated in the same menu. Again, it should be emphasized that for those elderly patients and cases of chronic consumptive diseases, the functions of the spleen-stomach, lungs and kidneys should be carefully protected. This point is crucial for the convalescence and rehabilitation of the sick.

F. Embodying the Body's Comprehensive Nutritional Needs

In biomedicine, it is stressed that the body needs all kinds of nutrients. This is similar to the idea in TCM, where dietotherapy embraces a macro and overall approach, which also embody the idea of modern nutriology. For instance, as early as in the *Huangdi's Internal Classic*, it had been emphasized that "for the health of the body, all kinds of cereals, fruits, flesh and vegetables should be taken." In the ancient Chinese classics, such as *Zhou Li* (*Rituals of the Zhou Dynasty*) and *Shi Jing* (*Classic of Poet*), it is mentioned that there are five crops, six crops, nine crops and even one hundred crops. Porridges made of all kinds of crops are the staple foods, which are of clinical significance. In TCM, porridges are believed to possess the potential to "nourish the spleen-stomach, replenish body fluids, regulate the spleen and strengthen the body's interior. It is good at dissipating edema and internal stuffiness and stimulating metabolism." *Ben Cao Gang Mu* (*Compendium of Materia Medica*) maintains that "morning porridge, which should be soft and tender in texture due to the empty stomach, is an excellent food." The wide varieties of porridge recorded in *Zhou Pa* (*Porridge Manual*) are still of great and practical significance even today. Since China is a country with vast territory, covering different climatic zones, crops ripen at different seasons and times, resulting in different natures, even of the same cereal. In dealing with crops for dietotherapy, the habits and food customs from different regions should also be addressed. Although some of the experts from Taoist and Buddhist sectors advocate vegetarian foods, they should not be treated as typical exponents for the ancient school of macrobiotics. In Sun Simiao's work on dietotherapy, as well as other works of the same sort, animal products are very common, including recipes containing flesh and milk from cows, mares, and wild animals as well. These reflect the ethnic features of national minorities, especially in the Tang and Yuan dynasties. It should be noted that China was the first to apply organotherapy, such as diabetes mellitus treated with pancreas, goiters treated with thyroid gland, strengthening of sexual function with external genitalia—all yielding satisfactory results. However, TCM stresses that such organotherapy should be strictly controlled to prevent over-dosage or prolonged administration, suggesting that TCM is aware of its side effect of hypofunction of the targeted organ. Furthermore, ancient Chinese also emphasized that vegetarian foods are essential and an integral part of dietotherapy. It is mentioned in *Zhou Li* (*Ritual of Zhou Dynasty*) that pears, hawthorns, Chinese dates, chestnuts, gourds and melons, and peaches are essential for daily life. Evidently, fruits and vegetables were recognized as essential and applied for dietotherapy. Again, TCM stresses the application of herbological theory when using vegetarian therapy, so that its mechanism can be brought into full play. For example, though oranges, tangerines and shaddocks are the same or similar sort of fruit, they still yield different actions. Tangerines have a red thin peel with pungent and bitter flavour and taste; oranges are a little bit larger and shaddocks are the largest with yellow and thick peel, which is pungent and sweet. All three are good at replenishing body fluid, stopping thirst, promoting urination, sobering excessive drinking, stimulating appetite (stomach), and expelling phlegm. However, modern scientific analysis claims that these three fruits yield different chemical constituents, i.e., shaddock is much more complicated and its therapeutic effects are also different. It has been proved that elements from shaddock peel are capable of anti-inflammation, anti-infection and anti-convulsion. Individual reports demonstrate that it also contains an insulin-type substance with glucose lowering capacity. Therefore, dietotherapy should not be based on traditional TCM theory alone; instead, modern biomedical knowledge should also share its contributions with TCM at the same time when administering dietotherapy.

G. Indications and Contraindications of Dietotherapy

Contraindications in dietotherapy have wide implications and coverage. Ingredients that conflict with one another should be carefully handled. When compounding a recipe for dietotherapy, this is a common rule. It is shown in *Huangdi's Internal Classic* that all tastes have their own preferential visceral affinity. For example, the crops of sour taste prefer the liver; bitter crops, the heart; sweet crops, the spleen; and salty crops, the kidneys. Also, all viscera have their own indications when they get sick. For example, for spleen diseases, rice, beef and Chinese dates are indicated; for heart diseases, wheat, mutton, apricots and Bulbus Allii Macrostemi; for lung diseases, yellow millet, chicken, peaches and Chinese onion; for liver diseases, sesame seeds, dog meat, plums and Chinese chives; and for kidney diseases, tender leaves of soybeans, pork, chestnuts and beans. Moreover, the *Internal Classic* also mentions contraindications of foods to the viscera, including avoidance of salty taste in heart diseases, pungent taste in liver diseases, sour taste in spleen diseases, bitter taste in lung diseases and sweet taste in kidney diseases. These are the basic theories of dietotherapy which are still of practical significance even nowadays. Over intake of a certain taste or flavour is also inappropriate. All these theories should be considered when providing dietotherapy, though further study is required by modern scientific approaches.

Contraindications in dietotherapy are also important. These include interactions among certain foods, and between foods and drugs as well. It is recorded in TCM literature that buckwheat, pork liver and soybean sauce mutually conflict, and should not be taken together; otherwise, former chronic diseases will relapse. In case pork liver is taken with fish, boils and carbuncles are apt to occur. Mutually antagonistic foods are also widely known, such as bee honey with raw Chinese onion and lettuce; soft-shell turtle with pork, armaranth, chicken egg, duck, or rabbit flesh; duck with walnut, fermented soy bean or edible fungi; Rhizoma Cur-culiginis with beef, cow's milk, etc. Controversies still persist over whether these contraindications from ancient literature are correct or not. Nevertheless, these allegedly conflicting foods should be taken into account when prescribing dietetic recipes. However, what Wang Shixiong of the Qing Dynasty said in his *Suixiju's Yin Shi Pu* (*Dietetic Menu*) is worthy of consideration and acceptance. He advocated that for cases of exuberant phlegm and fire with depletion of body fluids, the patient should avoid ginger, Chinese prickly ash and mutton. He said these are warm and dry and apt to aggravate or deteriorate the illness. Patients with exogenous infections not yet cured and those just recovering from ulcers, eye and throat diseases, smallpox or measles should avoid mustard, garlic, crab and hen's egg, all of which are apt to arouse endogenous evil-wind. Those with exuberant damp-heat should avoid taking foods encouraging damp and inflaming fire, such as malt sugar, bee honey, pork, sugar, cheese and butter. For cases of deficient spleen and interior cold, serious illness, and postpartum, foods, such as watermelons, plums, river snails, crab and clam, are apt to injure the body interior, abet cold evil and are contraindicated. Patients with massive bleeding, hemorrhoids and gestation should eschew pepper and arrowheads that deteriorate bleeding. Obviously, Wang's recommendations are easy to understand and acceptable, and also in line with the TCM idea of food contraindications. These are guiding principles for compounding dietotherapeutic recipes.

Contraindication of foods, when one is ill, refers to avoidance or restraint of consumption of those foods that are apt to arouse untoward or adverse reactions. Superficially, this seems similar to dietotherapy. Individuals from a community, when contract the same illness, may reveal quite different reactions to the same foods. An individual suffering from a certain disorder may be incompatible or contraindicated to some food, while another patient suffering from exactly the same illness may be contraindicated to other foods, but compatible to those unacceptable to the former. In addition, contraindications of food may change in the same individual at different stages of a disease. For example, at the hyperpyrexia stage of measles, ulcers or smallpox, it is natural that all foods inflaming evil-fire are contraindicated. Nevertheless, when the ulcers rupture or measles and smallpox transform into a convalescent stage, tonic foods believed to be "fermentable" are not contradicted but encouraged. The reason is that these are then essential and conducive to the recovery of the body. Contrarily, since the principles of dietotherapy are based on herbological theories, from which all contraindications of dietotherapy derived, these principles should be adhered to. In traditional Chinese dietotherapy, it is recorded that those cases violating the traditional regulations of contraindication are vulnerable to "dieto-relapse," due to immoderate meals, especially greasy and "fermentable" foods.

All in all, besides indications for dietotherapy, one should bear in mind the dietotherapeutic contraindications so as to accelerate the recovery when one falls ill.

IV. Varieties of Medicinal Foods

All human food, except for a few minerals, comes from the biological kingdom, including plants and animals, and are vulnerable to the natural process of fermentation or even putrefaction. To prevent these undesired phenomena and processes, and to meet the special demands relating to habits and customs of different communities, foods are processed into a great varieties of form, appearance and tastes with different nutritional values. These are termed foodstuffs, which fall under two categories; i.e., traditionally processed and present-day-processed foodstuffs. In the former group, foodstuffs are processed and compounded with medicines under the guidance of TCM theories, among others, together with herbological theories, termed medicinal foodstuffs or therapeutic foodstuffs which possess therapeutic or health-care actions with favourable colours, flavours, tastes and appearance. Ancient Chinese were aware that medical diets could prevent and treat diseases, as well as allow them to pursue longevity through medicinal diets. In the numerous "diet, dish, porridge, and tea" menus from the imperial palaces of successive ages, the folk masses, and medical works as well, a great variety of medicinal foods are recorded. The making of wines and spirits and leaven appeared as early as the 22nd century B.C., and were applied for treating stomach diseases in 597 B.C. In the earliest extant medical classic, *Huangdi's Internal Classic*, is a special chapter devoted to "Decoction, Liquid and Its Derivatives." Also, dietotherapeutic recipes are recorded, including "Decoction of Glutinous Rice and Pinellia," "Liquid of Chicken Dung," etc. These may be viewed as the first of their kind in the history of dietotherapeutic recipes. On the basis of summarizing various flavours and processing techniques from all parts of China during the development of history, these types of medicinal diets were greatly augmented and gradually completed. In *Shi Yi Xin Jian* (*Mirror of Dietotherapy*) of the Tang Dynasty, many sorts of medicinal foods, such as porridge, soups, liquids, cakes, juices, powders and a variety of dishes were included. In the Song Dynasty, *Tai Ping Sheng Hui Fang* (*Benevolent Recipe of Taiping Period*) and *Sheng Ji Zong Lu* (also *A Complete Collection of Holy Benevolence*) further augmented the contents of dietotherapy to include cheese, butter, puddings, pizza cakes, *yuntun* and many others. In the Ming and Qing dynasties, new varieties were added. For instance, in *Ben Cao Gang Mu* (*Compendium of Materia Medica*), steamed rice was subdivided into newly made steamed rice, ritual steamed rice, steamed rice of *hanshi* (eating-cool), etc. It also divided *gao* (puddings) into two groups: *shi* and *er*. The former can be made with steamed glutinous rice powder, millet powder and vulgare rice powder to form a paste; the latter can be prepared with mixed steamed powder of soybean, sugar plus honey.

By combining modern sorting methods with ancient literary records, modern medicinal diets can be classified as follows:

A. Based on Its Therapeutic Effects

This class is the common one applied in ancient medical literature. In *Shi Yi Xin Jian* (*Mirror of Dietotherapy*), the medicinal diets are classified into 15 kinds, each of which includes porridge, thick soup, dishes, liquids, etc. The 160 recipes in the relevant chapter of *Tai Ping Sheng Hui Fang* (*The Peaceful Holy Benevolent Prescription*) are divided into 28 kinds, each of which also includes porridge, thick soup, cake and liquids. A total of 29 kinds of recipes appears in *Sheng Ji Zong Lu*, each of which includes steamed rice, porridge, liquids, decoctions and honey paste.

In summary, therapeutically medicinal diets are divided into four categories:

(a) For health care: Mainly for weak and infirm people, who have no complaints. It is also applicable to normal people to promote health, prolong life and for cosmetic purposes.

(1) For slimming: Wax gourd plus chicken shreds with Radix Astragali seu Hedysari and ginseng; three peels processed with salt, slimming fermented glutinous rice, etc.

(2) For cosmetic purpose: Bamboo shoot plus sea cucumber, soft-shelled turtle soup with artemisia, bamboo shoot with finger-citron, bean curd with Chinese taro.

(3) For intelligence-promotion: Brain improving porridge, honey-

processed preserved fruits for intelligence, yam plus snakehead, siliquose pelvetia plus calamus.

(4) For strength: Ginseng plus pigeon, thick soup of yam plus bean curd and sealwort.

(5) For promoting sight: Sheep liver plus Flos Buddlejae, chrysanthemum drink plus Semen Cassiae; pheasant plus Semen Cellosia.

(6) For promoting hearing: Pig kidney with Fructus Corni and powdered Radix Puerariae.

(7) For healthy teeth: Green tea with Herba Dendrobii, marrow porridge plus Herba Portulacae, duck of eight-ingredients for nourishing the kidneys and consolidating teeth.

(8) For hair: Fruit gel for hair, rice pudding with three beans for blackening hair, honey preserved fruit for replenishing blood and hair, carrots with Radix Polygonati Multiflori.

(9) For weight gain: Sandwich cake with Poria, chicken with chestnut and Bulbus Lilli.

(10) For prolonging life: Immortal's porridge, life-prolonging gelatin.

(b) For prevention of illness: Grass carp with Chinese onion and ginger for influenza, cherry with glycyrrhizae and preserved fruit for pharyngitis, green bean soup for heat stroke and diarrhoea, purslance for dysentery, etc.

(c) For treatment:

(1) For infection of the superficies: Sugar and ginger drink, decoction of Allii Fistulosi and Sojae Preparation with millet wine.

(2) For expectoration, short breath and cough: Anti-cough paste of pear.

(3) For improving digestion: Sugar-tea paste for digestion, pork chop with nuts, dry pork with hawthorn, spleen-invigorating cake.

(4) For antipyresis or clearing heat: Tomato and watermelon juice, five-ingredient juice, fresh drink of seven ingredients.

(5) For expelling cold: Mutton with aconitum, mutton with Radix Angelica Sinensis and ginger, lichee porridge.

(6) For eliminating dampness: Steamed bread with Semen Myristica, stuffed steamed bread with poria.

(7) For catharsis: Honey with sesame oil, potato honey paste.

(8) For tonification: Cooked hen with Radix Angelica Simensis and ginseng, duck with cordyceps, rooster steamed seven times.

(9) For regulating *qi*: Duck with clove, chicken with Pericarpium Citri Reticulata.

(10) For regulating blood circulation: Decoction of Chinese dates and ginseng, chicken with Radix Angelica Sinenesis, beef jelly.

(11) For calming down wind: Flesh slices with chrysanthemum, fish head with Rhizoma Gastrodiae.

(12) For sedation: Porridge of Semen Ziziphi spinosae, decoction of onion and dates.

(d) For convalescence: During the process of convalescence, the functions or internal organs are in a *qi*-deficiency state. The medicaments mostly applied include ginseng and Radix Astragali seu Hedysari crystals, cream of Radix Angelica Sinensis, ginseng and yam (Radix Dioscorea). Because of conditions of deficiency of the blood and its *yin* component, malnutrition of the viscera may lead to further blood deficiency; hence, baked sheep heart with rose, fresh longan immersed in sugar and thick soup of pork skin with dates are indicated. Furthermore, convalescent cases used to have an exuberance of *yang* component due to *yin* deficiency, eventually resulting in deficiencies of both *yin* and *yang*. Thus, replenishing *yin* to clear away inner heat is needed. The medicinal diets include decoction of crystal sugar with Rhizoma Polygonati, malt sugar, etc. Conversely, when disharmony appears due to deficient *yang* component, invigoration of *yang* is needed. The medicinal food may include cooked mutton and stewed chicken cubes with Rhizoma Alpiniae officinalis. In case of a shortage or depletion of body fluid, supplement of this fluid is essential. Medicinal diets for this disorder include spirit of fats with Chinese dates and honey paste of longan and ginseng. Deficiencies of *yin* component, fluid, blood, as well as *yang* component, can occur after a serious illness. At this time, imbibition of a variety of tonics which are not dry and greasy is recommended. Common medicinal diets include black beans, apricot kernels, and steamed glutinous rice with eight-ingredients.

B. Classified by Processing Methods

It is not unusual that in ancient Chinese medical literature medicinal foods are classified on the basis of their processing technique. In *Yang Lao Feng Qin Shu* (*The Book of Taking Care of Parents and Elderly*) of the Song Dynasty, four kinds of medicinal diets are distinguished, i.e., soft food, solid food, drinks, and dishes, each including various subgroups. Meanwhile *Zun Sheng Ba Qian* (*Eight Discourses on Macrobiotice*) of the Ming Dynasty gives 10 kinds of medicinal diets; namely, tea of spring, soup, boiled drinks, fruit and powder, meat and fish, vegetables, brewed food, sweet food, porridge and processed medicine. A modern text on medicinal diet, *Practical TCM Nutriology*, classifies medicinal diets into the following categories: Steamed rice and porridge, cake and pastry, soup and thick soup, juice and drink, paste and liquid. Therefore, it can be summarized that medicinal diets are of the following types:

Fresh juice This is made from juicy rhizomes, leaves, stems or fruits by first grating and then squeezing. A suitable amount of water or wine can be added. In ancient times, such fresh juices from watermelons, pears and tomatoes were used for thirst due to febrile diseases, while juices from fresh lotus leaves or root were used in bleeding due to fever. Juices from turnips were used to promote digestion and resolve phlegm.

Tea drinking Substances, with or without tea, are grated as coarse powder. No cooking is needed, but only immersion with boiling water is enough. This is an old form of medicinal food; for instance, ginger, a tea drink, is recorded in *Sheng Ji Zong Lu* (*General Collection for Holy Relief*) of the Song Dynasty.

Decoction This is prepared by boiling the substance in water, or simply by immersing it in water and then discarding the residue. This is one of the oldest forms of medicinal food. However, the useful portion of the residue can also be eaten. When the substances are rare or valuable, they may be prepared by stewing or steaming. Common examples: Decoction of Chinese onion and dates from Qian Jin Fang for neurasthenia; decoction of lotus seeds and six-in-one ingredients from Ren Zhai Zhi Zhi Fang for urinary infection; and decoction of double lotus from *Tai Ping Sheng Hui Fang* for gastrointestinal bleeding.

Instant drinks This form of food is made from dry materials which are first boiled and then filtered. Fresh juice may also be used. The residue is discarded and the solution is then further concentrated by boiling.

After concentration, dry sugar powder or binder is added to form granules which are then dried. A solution is made by adding boiling water. Examples include instant powder of Herba seu Radix Cirsii Japonici and

Herba Cephelanoploris for all bleedings, and instant powder of glycyrrhiza and tangerine for pharyngitis and laryngitis.

Medicinal Spirits These are further divided into Jiu, Li and Liao. Jiu is a transparent solution of distilled spirits immersed with medicines, such as Fructus Lycii spirits and Fructus Chaenomelis spirits. Li is a solution of spirits plus sugar, such as Li of red bayberry for preventing summer heat and Li of Cortex Acanthopanacis Radicis for strengthening tendons and bones. Liao is prepared by adding distilled grains (residue), such as Semen Coicis Liao for resolving dampness, strengthening spleen and improving appearance and chrysanthemum Liao for vertigo due to hypertension of liver heat type.

Syrup Also called Fang Xiang Shui (aromatic water). This is a kind of aromatic plant, prepared by vapour distillation to form a volatile, oily or watery solution. Syrup first appeared in the Yuan Dynasty. In *Ben Cao Gang Mu Shi Yi (Supplement of Compendium of Materia Medica)*, there is over a score of syrups listed, such as rose and jasmine. Nowadays, the common syrups include loquat for moistening the lung and stopping coughs, apricot nut syrup for anti-asthma, and syrup of Flos Lonicerae for clearing away evil heat.

Honey paste This is a kind of sticky paste prepared by boiling foods with medicines and then concentrated after residue is discarded and sugar or honey added. This forms a condensed paste which is served as a tonic with moistening potential. It is indicated for the infirm and chronic cases for long-term administration. Traditional honey pastes still in use include honey paste of autumn pear for coughing of lung-heat type, hair-blackening honey paste of *jishantangs*, and Jing Yan Fang (Empirical Recipe) for premature white hair or hair loss.

Porridge This can be prepared from starchy cereals, including rice, millet, glutinous rice, wheat or barley, by slow cooking. Medicinal porridge is prepared by adding medicines to regular porridge. The ancient Chinese felt that porridges were especially helpful for the elderly and the infirm, as well as for postpartum problems and post-illness. Common medicinal porridges include red-bean porridge with Cagongrass root from *Zhou Hou Bei Ji Fang* for edema, and sheep's kidney porridge with fruit of Chinese wolfberry from *Sheng Ji Zong Lu* for pain in the waist, knees and heels.

Powder This is the dry end product of foods, rich in starch after hydrolysis by frying, steaming or cooking to form a dry cream powder with dextrin and sugar. The cream can be taken simply by adding water to form a paste. The common ones include lotus root powder, water chestnut powder, powder of oily flour, and apricot nut powder.

Broth A thick soup prepared by boiling meat, egg, milk or seafood. Medicinal broth is formed by adding drugs of neutral or plain nature (taste). Examples of ancient broth still in use today are finless-eel broth with Radix Angelica Sinensis and ginseng for invigorating strength, *qi* and blood; pig trotter brother for promoting lactation during postpartum, and meat broth with yam and milk as a tonic for the infirm.

Candy This is the solid or semisolid state of sugar after boiling with water. Medicinal candy is prepared by adding crude powder of drugs into boiled sugar. Traditional candy still used today includes clove-ginger candy for vomiting, hiccupe due to cold in stomach from Zhai Yuan Fang; candy of persimmon powder from dry persimmon surface for dry coughing due to hot-lung and dry pharynx from *Sui Xi Ju Menu*; digestive candy for promoting digestion, a popular folk recipe, and anti-cough candy of pear paste for common colds of exogenous causes.

Preserved fruit or honey-prepared food These are prepared by immersing fruits or other foods in honey or sugar. For medicinal use, it is preserved with food, sugar, honey and drug mixed together. The common ones include preserved hawthorn, preserved peach, preserved plum and preserved tangerine peel.

Food made of flour and rice This is prepared from rice, glutinous rice, flour as steamed rice, pudding, cake, and rolls, all of which can be prepared by boiling, steaming, baking, frying, or serving cool. When drugs are added to these foods, the dish becomes medicinal rice or flour food. The drugs used are mostly of neutral nature. Traditional ones still in use today include poria cake, cake of eight ingredients, kidney-bean roll, cake of tangerine peel, steamed rice with ginseng and Chinese red date.

Dishes This refers to dishes made of vegetable, meat, egg, milk or seafood by various cooking techniques. Medicinal dishes are prepared with relevant drugs in lovely colour, appearance and attractive smell. A great variety of medicinal dishes are available, such as carp with Chinese onion and ginger, duck with cordyceps, chicken with *Radix Astragali seu Hedysari*, and fish with Chinese toon, etc.

Miscellaneous There are many medicinal foods that do not fall under the above categories, such as sesame-salt powder, spicy areca, medicinal black bean, etc.

C. Based on the Nature of Source Materials

This category can be divided into the following: Cereals, vegetables, fruits, meat from birds and beasts, seafoods, eggs and milk. In *Yin Shi Bian Lu* (*Record of Differentiation for Foods*), there are 39 kinds of substances which serve as a type of tea, including juice from roots, rhizomes, leaves, flowers and fruits. These produce turnip juice, plum juice, wax gourd juice, etc. Under the category of cereal are 53 kinds of porridge and 32 types of spirits.

As history evolves, medicinal foods also change and improve as advanced techniques are applied. Nowadays, cans of blood tonic, strengthening aerated water and chest-easing cola are available, as well as many others of the same sort, all with Chinese dietotherapeutic features.

V. The Range of Medicinal Foods

A wide range of medicinal foods are currently available for therapeutic use, health care and daily life:

A. For Therapeutic Application

In prehistoric society, food was used either alone or together with drugs for treating diseases. Medicinal food is the combination of food with treatment remedies. Numerous materials of dietotherapy are recorded in ancient Chinese medical literature. Instances include *Shang Han Lun* (*Treatise on Febrile Disease*) and *Bei Ji Qian Jing Yao Fang* (*Prescriptions Worth Thousand Gold for Emergencies*). In the former, soup of pork skin for sore throat due to asthenic heat is described, as well as soup of mutton with Radix Angelica Sinensis for postpartal abdominal pain and cold hernia with anemia; in the latter, we find carp soup for dampness in the uterus of a pregnant woman.

For application in the treatment of diseases, dietotherapy should be administered in accordance with different individuals, places and seasons.

Administering Dietotherapy

Importance of pinpointing its uses:

The constitution of each individual varies just as his or her facial appearance. Likewise, each individual has his own preference for and reaction to different foods. For instance, some people like spicy foods or strong-smelly preserved bean curd, while others detest it. Milk is a common drink to some, while to others it may cause diarrhoea. Cucumbers are a very common food to most of us; however, it may cause allergic reactions in some individuals, producing abdominal pain, diarrhoea, vomiting or even fever.

An individual's constitution may be classified as cold, hot, deficient or excessive. Generally speaking, an individual with a deficient constitution, featuring a thin body, sallow or pale complexion, with short breath, etc., should take more nutritious food; this would not be necessary for those individuals with an excessive constitution. Strangely enough, some deficient individuals simply cannot accept nourishing foods, which only cause them discomfort; they can only take common or plain foods. For those with a hot constitution, hot and dried foods made by frying, baking or roasting, as well as spicy foods should be avoided. Certain individuals can stand up to one pound of longan or lichee without any reaction, while others suffer from epistaxis (nose bleeds) after having eaten only ten pieces. A fat person is said to have a high phlegm and wet constitution and should take more foods which are plain and easily digested, whereas thin people are said to be deficient and should take more nourishing foods for replenishing fluids. In brief, dietotherapy quite obviously should be administered according to the needs and constitutions of different individuals and should never be applied indiscriminately.

Seasonal changes are another important factor in the application of dietotherapy. Medicinal foods should vary according to the different seasons. For instance, during the hot summer months, it is not feasible to prescribe a diet of a dry, hot or greasy nature; instead, plain, cool and non-greasy foods are preferable. On cold winter days, however, nourishing paste or even a little greasy food is recommended. According to the traditional view, even the food eaten at specific times within a single day should vary. It is advisable to take easily digested, non-greasy, yet nutritious food, for breakfast, and greasy and nourishing food for lunch. It is highly advisable not to take greasy food or food difficult to digest at dinner. After an early dinner, eat no more prior to going to bed, or sleep will be disturbed.

However, it should be stressed that the above rules are summarized from the long experience of the Chinese; as a result, they are recommended for peoples of other regions and countries in principle only. These precepts should not be used stereotypically. The physical constitutions, geographical conditions and climates in other places of the world are not always the same as those of China. However, the above principles are all applicable to people of all ethnic groups and countries as long as they are used in accordance with their own concrete conditions.

Geographical conditions are also important. For instance, China is a vast country; when the northern part is still deeply frozen, the southern portion is already blooming with colour. For northern inhabitants, nourishing pastes or slightly greasy foods, even foods of a hot nature, are permissible. For southerners, foods of a cold nature and those easily digested, rather than greasy foods, are preferred. Moreover, inhabitants in different parts of the country have widely different habits regarding food and drink. Some prefer pungent and spicy foods, while others prefer sour, sweet or salty diets. It all depends on the climatic and geographical conditions which lead to the development of habits and customs over many generations. Investigations should be made at the time the therapy is carried out, so as to avoid incompatibility and troubles due to neglect of differences in climate, habits or personal physical constitutions.

B. For Health Care Promotion

Medicinal foods, as one of the many measures for the health care of humankind, have a coverage much wider than for therapeutic purposes. Nowadays, foods for health care are mostly tonics and nutritious foods of natural sources rather than chemically synthesized. Habitually, these tonics are not served as staple or nonstaple foods. Not a few medicinal foods fall under the category of promoting health care.

(1) Nutritious nourishing food

It is estimated that about one-tenth of the herbs in TCM pharmacology are for nourishing, i.e., about 500 kinds of herbs, mostly recognized through long-term experiences, with a part manufactured by modern processing techniques. The common ones are ginseng, cordyceps, Radix Astragali seu Hedysari, yam, Radix Atractylodis Macrocephalae, Rhizoma Gastrodiae, poria, glycyrrhizae, Radix Angelica Sinensis, Radix Polygoni Multiflori, Rhizoma Polygonati, walnuts, sesame seeds, Chinese red or black dates, swallow's nest, soft-shell turtle, lotus seed, Job's tears, honey, white fungus, and dry longan. Modern processing products, such as royal jelly with ginseng, as well as those recorded in ancient books, are all conducive to the health of the elderly and the infirm. These include decoction of ginseng and dates and Jiva's decoction (composed of butter, ginger, seeds of Chinese chive in distilled spirits, honey, sesame seeds, cinnamon leaves, prepared soybeans and crude sugar). These all help replenish blood and invigorate *qi* and *yang*, as well as moisten actions of the bowel. There is another "pork kidney spirits" of the Qing Dynasty for lumbago and hypofunction of the kidney. These spirits are prepared by placing a pair of pig kidneys immersed in 2 cups of infantile urine and a cup of spirits. Transfer this to a pot and seal tightly with mud. Cook the pot with a small fire in the evening until dawn. The food is then ready for serving. A so-called "Xia Jiren's Recipe" of the Tang Dynasty is a beauty remedy composed of apricot nut and sheep fat, while the "Mastaji Soup" of the Yuan Dynasty is made up of mutton, Cortex Cinnamomi, Huihui beans, fragrant rice and Mastaji spicy, which is a medicinal food for nourishing and warming the body interior. A recipe of the Ming Dynasty, "Cake of Rhizome Polygonati," is prepared by mixing the rhizome with soybean and sugar. This is a tonic for nourishing and clearing the lung. An "Orange Cake" of the Qing Dynasty, prepared by mixing orange peel, plum, glycyrrhiza and sandlewood, is beneficial for nourishing fluid, eliminating stagnation, expelling bad odor, resolving phlegm and regulating the spleen and stomach. Another recipe, "Wang Ling Paste," is made up of longan and Western ginseng; it is a strong tonic for blood and *qi* without aggravating the pre-existing inner evil fire.

(2) Dishes for health care

Foods made of medicine and prepared for health promotion are plentiful, including dishes, appetizers, snacks, sweets and honey-preserved fruits. Cooking processes are again multifarious, including steaming, frying, brothing, cooking, boiling, dry frying, slow boiling, immersing, smoking and salt-preserving. In addition, special cooking techniques can also be utilized. For example, honey plum-blossom, and lotus root stuffed with pomegranate powder. The latter is made by filling the spaces in the lotus root with pomegranate powder and then steaming the food together. Again, "Cooked-Pear Recipe" is prepared by filling the small foramen in a pear with Chinese prickly ash; then wrap the pear with flour and stew it until well-done.

Beverages for promoting health also come in various types, including soups, drinks, spirits, milk, tea, juice, syrup and thick liquids. For different types of tea, in *Yin Shan Zheng Yao* are found recipes for Chinese wolfberry tea, Western tea and Sichuan tea. As for a variety of milks, these come from humans, cows, sheep, and mares, as well as butter and cheese. For syrup, plants rich in fluid such as cereals, vegetables, fruits, gourds, grasses, flowers and leaves are squeezed and fresh juice obtained for distillation. It is claimed that syrup is an excellent moistener and antipyretic remedy. The common ones in use are syrup of honeysuckle and syrup of wolfberry bark. Juices are obtained from fresh fruits and vegetables, such as sugar cane and reed rhizome. A common juice called "Five-Ingredient Drink" is made up of juices from sugar cane, pear, reed rhizome, fresh water chestnut and fresh lotus root. The solution is made by cooking. "Ginseng Solution of Three Ingredients" is prepared by decocting ginseng with dry longan, lotus seeds, and Chinese dates. "Qiju Drink" is prepared by cooking chrysanthemum with fruit of Chinese wolfberry. Many tonic-spirits or health-promoting medicinal spirits are also applied in daily use, including Shenji Spirits, which is a fruit of Chinese wolfberry with ginseng, immersed in spirits. Other spirits include cordycep, plum-blossom and chrysanthemum spirits. "Overall Tonic of Ten Ingredients" and "Xuanju Solution" (made of ants in spirits) are both strong tonics.

C. For Daily Application

Medicinal foods can greatly enrich the fullness of daily life by improving the physical constitution and is widely applied. Diets featuring Chinese national uniqueness are now attracting increasing interest worldwide.

The advent of medicinal food in modern banquets or feasts is of significance. Chinese medicinal foods have a long history and are rich in variety. Traditionally, they emphasized their therapeutic aspects, and had not yet been popularly accepted by the masses in their daily lives. Over the years people endeavoured to change this condition. They combined traditional dietotherapeutic theory and practice with modern nutriological achievements to prepare medicinal banquets to promote health. As a result, these medicinal banquets and feasts have now come into being. Such banquets are character-ized by palatable tastes devoid of drug smell, but with attractive appearance and full of cultural dietary flavour.

Modernization of traditional medicinal diets. Due to its many advantages, including its easy and acceptable method of administration, Chinese dietoth-erapy is now widely popular in China and among oversea Chinese. Increas-ingly, people in other countries have also become interested in Chinese medicinal diets. However, due to the inconvenience of food processing for medicinal purposes, the forms of medicinal foods have undergone a reforma-tion so as to ensure easy administration. There are many common new forms of modern medicinal foods, including canned foods, snacks, all kinds of aerated drinks, confectionaries, instant powder or granules and many others, all made by modern processing techniques for easy transportation, storage and administration. Of course, the original therapeutic and medicinal features should be just as well-preserved as those served in the more traditional way. Integration of traditional medicinal food with modern science and techniques will certainly bring even more promising prospects to dietotherapy in the future.

VI. Special Foods for Common Medical Problems

As mentioned above, one of the unique elements of traditional Chinese medicine is the basing of its treatment on the differential diagnosis of symptoms and signs. The nature of the disease, either deficient or excessive, cold or hot, superficial or interior, should first be determined and treatment then given on the basis of such diagnosis. The process for dietotherapy is the same. Below are some of the medicinal foods recommended for certain common medical problems.

A. Internal Problems

1. Common cold

In traditional Chinese medicine, common cold is divided into two types, cold-wind and hot-wind, which should be treated with different medicinal foods.

Cold-wind type: Manifestations are fever, chilliness without perspiration, headache, pains over the whole body, obstruction of nose (stuffy nose), nasal secretion (runny nose), white coated tongue, mildly quick pulse.

Prescriptions:

a. Decoction of ginger with sugar: 25 g of ginger, cleaned and sliced into small chips, then put into a bowl. Add boiling water and cover for 5-10 minutes. Add an equal amount (25 g) of brown sugar. Drink the decoction while hot, then cover up well, sleep and start to sweat.

b. Decoction of scallion and ginger: Scallion stalk and fresh ginger, 25 g each. Cut into small pieces. Prepare a small bowl of bean starch vermicelli, or rice or flour noodles with salt. Add the scallion and ginger pieces and eat. Then cover up well, sleep and start to sweat.

Hot-wind type: Manifestations are high fever, no chilliness, slight sweating, red eyes, sore throat, headache, slightly yellow coated tongue and rapid pulse.

Prescriptions:

a. Chrysanthemum, peppermint and mulberry leaf drink: Chrysanthemum and mulberry leaves, 5 g each, bitter bamboo leaves and cogon root, 30 g each, and peppermint, 3 g. Put all the ingredients in a bowl or cup, pour in boiling water and cover for 10 minutes. Drink the decoction like tea.

b. Peppermint sweets: Boil 500 g cane sugar with a considerable amount of water at a low heat until it becomes sticky. Then slowly add 5 ml peppermint powder or peppermint oil and stir steadily until the mixture sticks to the stirring implement like threads. Pour the sugar into a big porcelain tray (coated with a thin layer of vegetable oil). Cut the hardened sugar into small pieces. Take several times daily for a mild common cold.

c. Decoction of scallion with fermented soybeans: Boil 10 g fermented soybeans in 200 ml water for 2-3 minutes. Then add 25 g scallion white bulbs sliced into small chips and serve. Drink the decoction and cover well for mild sweating.

d. Stir-fried chilli with fermented soybeans: Stir-fry separately chilli and fermented soybeans, each 250 g. Then mix them together and add some salt. This is a tasty dish and can be served for regular meals as side dish, especially for porridge.

e. Cold turnip slivers: Cut 500 g turnip into fine slivers. Add some sesame oil, salt and monosodium glutamate and serve as a side dish. No vinegar should be added. This is especially good for cases with profuse sputum excretion.

2. Influenza (flu)

Generally known as "severe common cold." Its manifestations are sudden onset, severe headache and pain over whole body, congestion of the eyes and throat, coughing and high fever. It is highly infectious, usually affecting many people in the same area.

Prescriptions:

a. Thoroughly rinse and clean 250 g turnip. Chop up then immerse in vinegar for several hours. Eat with hot rice porridge.

b. Take soybeans, 10 g, and fresh coriander, 30 g. Cook the soybeans in water for about 15-20 minutes, then add the coriander and boil for another 10 minutes. Eat the whole dose once daily.

c. Take tender peppermint leaves, 3 g, and licorice root, 3 g. Put them together in a cup, pour in boiling water and cover for 15 minutes. Drink it hot, two or three times a day.

d. Take bean curd, 200 g, processed (fermented) soybeans, 12 g, and scallion stalk, 15 g. Cook bean curd in water until it is well done. Add fermented bean and scallion stalk and boil for another 20 minutes. Eat it all while hot, then cover up well, sleep and sweat slightly.

3. Bronchitis

This refers to chronic bronchitis, not acute bronchitis developing from a common cold, which is the result of long irritation of the bronchus. Its manifestations are coughing with sputum and with no, or very mild, fever or headache.

a. Take a reasonable amount of rock candy and a pear, about 200 g, chopped into pieces. Put these two in a bowl or cup, and steam in a water both for half an hour. Eat the whole dose once or twice a day for 1-2 weeks.

b. Pig's lung porridge: Take a whole pig's lung of about 500 g, rinse and bring to boil. After skimming, boil for another half an hour, then remove the pig's lung and chop. Mix some of the soup and 100 g chopped lung with 100 g rice and 50 g seed of Job's-tears, cooking gently until soup becomes glutinous, rice and lung well done. Add some salt, ginger, onion or other spices and serve. This porridge is good for chronic cough, emaciation, profuse sputum or sputum with blood.

c. Lily porridge: Take dried lily 30 g (or 60 g fresh lily), a reasonable amount of rock candy and rice, 100 g. Boil the lily first for 15 minutes, then add the rice and cook at a low heat until it becomes glutinous. Add the rock candy and boil for a further short while.

This porridge is good for moistening the lungs and is indicated for chronic bronchitis. It is not suitable for acute common cold, or acute bronchitis.

d. Nuts preserved with honey: Boil 250 g stir-fried sweet apricot nuts in water for about an hour. Add 250 g walnuts. Boil until almost dry, then pour in 500 g honey, stirring continuously. Remove from heat as soon as it boils.

This preserved medicinal sweet is good for general body weakness, and bronchitis with prolonged coughing and shortness of breath.

4. Infectious hepatitis

Remarks: For patients with hepatitis, the diets should be based on the conditions of the hepatic functions. Food poisonous to the liver should be strictly avoided. Spirits, liquor and wine of any kind, including beer, are totally forbidden. Animal fats from pork, beef or mutton should be limited, because the digestion of fats increases the work of the liver. Proteins, either animal or vegetables, protect the liver cells and should be taken in suitable amount. Excessive intake of protein, especially at the acute stage, produces much metabolites toxic to the liver. Hence, it can only be taken properly. Vitamins are also essential to the function of liver.

Apart from those with biliary stones or hemolytic jaundice, those icteric patients with low fever can be treated by this method.

a. Vinegar and bone soup: Take 100 ml of vinegar (best prepared from glutinous rice), fresh pig's bone (best vertebrae), 500 g, and brown and white sugar, 125 g each.

Smash up the bones with a hammer and immerse in the vinegar. Add both sugars and then boil for half an hour. After it has cooled, filter with gauze. Discard the residue and keep the strained liquid in a bottle. Administer according to different ages:

5-10 years   10-15 ml.
11-15 years   20-30 ml.
adults   30-40 ml.

Three times daily after meals, one month for a course. Interrupt a week before another course begins. For chronic hepatitis, 2-3 courses may be needed.

b. Loach powder: Keep several live loaches in fresh water for 1-2 days to rid them of impurities. Bake in an oven at 100°C until dry. If one has no oven, it may be boiled then dried over a stove. Grind into powder. Dosage: 10 g, three times a day. For children the dose may be reduced. One course lasts 12-16 days. For chronic patients, several courses may be needed.

c. River snail soup: Put 10-20 live river snails in fresh water for 1-2 days so they evacuate any internal impurities. Crack the shells and take out the flesh. Mix with a cup of yellow rice wine, then dilute with water and cook. Drink the soup, though the flesh can also be eaten. Take once daily for a period according to the reaction.

d. Chinese date porridge: Rinse 10-20 Chinese dates. Cook 100 g of rice, adding the dates when the water comes to the boil and simmer until it becomes a glutinous porridge. It should be eaten daily over an extended period. If Chinese dates are not available, 30 g of Chinese wolfberry seeds may serve as a substitute, prepared in the same way.

e. Five-Juice Drink: Rinse the following fruits and vegetables: pear, water chestnut, lotus root, each 100 g; Radix Ophipogonis, 50 g; fresh Rhizome Phragmitis, 100 g. Grind into small pieces. Squeeze out juice. Drink suitable amount of the juice for 5-7 days.

f. Steamed fish with vinegar and sugar: Take 500 g of black carp with scales and inner viscera discarded. Put it on a dish with some ginger filaments over the fish and inside its body. Steam it for 10-15 minutes. Then heat some vegetable oil with some water to which vinegar and white sugar are added. Add some corn starch. Continue to heat until the solution becomes sticky. Pour it onto the fish and serve.

5. Mumps (parotitis)

A kind of viral infection in which the salivary glands, mainly the parotic gland, are affected. Its manifestations are swellings and pain at the subaural region, especially during mastication. Sometimes, when not well treated, the sexual glands, especially the testes, may be adversely effected, even resulting in sterility.

a. Soak 50 g of red beans in water for 1-2 hours. A portion is then pounded in a mortar and applied locally. The rest of the beans should be well-cooked and eaten. It should be taken at each meal for one week or until the illness is cured.

b. Rinse 50 g of fresh (or 20 g dry) day-lily and soak in water for half an hour, then bring to boil and simmer for 20 minutes. Take all the day-lily and soup, once daily.

c. Thick soup of balsam pear: Rinse 2 pieces of balsam pear and pound it to form a paste. Mix some salt and stir thoroughly. Discard the residues after half an hour and boil it with a little corn (or sweet potato) starch to make a semi-transparent thick soup. Drink the soup in several parts.

Remarks: I myself suffered from bilateral parotitis at the age of 24 with a high fever of 39°C, swelling, pain and hot subauricular region. Pain was so severe that chewing was very difficult. This thick soup was administered on the third day. On the next day, fever and tender parts greatly subsided and I was able to take some semifluid meals. The illness was totally cured 2 days later with no complications.

6. Dysentery

Remarks: A patient came to visit me, complaining of repeated attacks of purulent diarrhoea for several months. There were 4-5 bowel movements each day. At that time, medicines were very scarce in the rural areas and no Western drugs were available at the moment. I made the diagnosis of chronic bacillary dysentery and prescribed fresh garlic, one bulb, twice a day. The patient took the garlic as ordered for one week and he was cured with normal stool appearance, with no more abdominal pain when defecating.

An observation reported several hundred dysentery cases, with a cured rate of over 95 percent. The temperature turned normal within 1-2 days, with tenesmus subsiding within 2-5 days on average. Stools were normal in 2-4 days, with no sequalae of constipation. It was reported that the garlic with purple peel yields better results than the white-peeled ones.

Dietotherapy alone should only be used in chronic cases. For acute cases, drug therapy should mainly be administered at the same time.

a. Green tea with honey: 5 g of green tea infused in boiling water and left to stand for 10 minutes. Add some honey and then drink before it is cold. Repeat 3-4 times daily.

b. Garlic: 10-15 g of fresh garlic, eaten either whole or crushed. Since it may irritate the mouth's mucous membrane, some other food may be taken at the same time. Generally, one head of garlic daily is enough. If taken crushed, 30-60 g of purslane may be first boiled to make a soup and then added. A little white sugar may also be added. Administer 1-2 times daily for half a month. The second course should be after one week's interruption.

c. Dark plum (Fructus Mume) decoction: Make a concentrated decoction with 5-6 pieces of dark plum. Best taken before meals. It can be prepared in paste form by boiling 5 kg of dark plum at a low heat until well done. Discard the stones and filter. Cook the filtrate until it becomes sticky. Then prepare it as bean-sized pills. Take 3-5 pills, twice daily.

d. Pomegranate peel: It shows a definite effect on chronic diarrhoea and dysentery. Rinse 20 g of pomegranate peel and boil it for thirty minutes. Add some brown sugar and then discard the residue. Drink one cupful, 2-3 times daily.

e. Turnip: Take 500 g of peeled turnip, rinse and slice. Add cane sugar and vinegar in adequate amount according to taste. Eat as you like at meals.

f. Decoction of dried persimmon and brown sugar: Dry 500 g dried persimmon over a low heat until scorched, then grind into powder and store in a bottle. Dosage: 10 g with some brown sugar, swallowed with warm water, twice daily. May be administered over an extended period.

g. Braised finless eel: 500 g live finless eel, cleaned and cut into slices. First fry it and then add a little soybean sauce, vinegar, garlic and brown sugar. Add a little water, ground ginger and starch. After starch becomes sticky, it is ready for serving.

h. Purslane decoction: Take 200 g fresh purslane (itself a tasty wild vegetable), 10-20 g hyacinth flower, and boil together for 15 minutes. The decoction can then be administered. Purslane may also be prepared in powdered form after drying. Take 5 g for each dose with sugar, twice daily.

7. Malaria

Acute malaria can be satisfactorily controlled by drugs, while for chronic cases, the following dieto-remedies are recommended.

a. Carambola drink: Squeeze 1 kg carambola. Cook the juice over a low heat until it becomes sticky. After this paste has cooled, add 500 g white sugar and store in a bottle. Dosage: 1 teaspoonful, thrice daily.

b. Wild duck soup: Prepare a wild duck of about 1 kg, discarding the viscera and feathers. Cook with several slices of ginger, dates, a little oil, salt and yellow rice wine. Eat the meat and drink the soup. May be eaten over 2 or more days. Effective for chronic malaria.

c. Soft-Shell Turtle Soup: A soft-shell turtle with shell and viscera removed is cut into cubes and cooked in a pot with some pig fat. Add some salt after well-done and eat in one meal.

d. Soup of Mutton and Soft-Shell Turtle: The turtle and mutton are cut into cubes and cooked together with slow fire. Add some sugar and salt. Take a small bowl of the flesh with soup.

Remarks: A 10-year-old boy, coming from southern China, visited our clinic. His chief complaint was irregular fever, general malaise and emaciation. He moved with his parents to northern China only 6 months before. His homeland is an area with high incidence of malaria. Two years ago, he suffered from regular fever with chilliness, once every other day. Though he received antimalarial remedy, he didn't complete a full course of treatment. Since then, he became weaker and weaker with irregular fever. Blood smear revealed positive malarial parasites. Soup of mutton and soft-shell turtle, together with 7 doses of qinghao (Artemisia Annua) were prescribed. He revisited our clinic 2 weeks later with apparent amelioration of general condition. Blood exams revealed no more parasites present. He was in good health 6 months later when he revisited the clinic for a general health checkup.

8. Iron-deficient anaemia

This is the commonest type of all anaemic disorders. The foods mentioned here are effective only for iron-deficient anaemia, not for other types.

a. Date and sheep's bone porridge. Take 1-2 crushed sheep tibial bones, and 20-30 pitted dates. Boil the bones for 1-2 hours over a slow heat. Make porridge with 100-200 g of rice and the dates. Mix these two and boil for a short time longer. This will make 2 or 3 doses. Take daily for half to one month.

b. Bean porridge with brown sugar. Take 100 g of glutinous rice, 20 pieces of Chinese dates, black beans, 30 g, and brown sugar in sufficient quantity. Boil the rice with the black beans until glutinous porridge is half prepared, then the pitted Chinese dates are added. The brown sugar is finally added once the porridge is ready. This can be eaten everyday over a long period.

c. Spinach and pig's liver soup. Take 100 g pig's liver, sliced, and 100 g spinach cut into segments. Coat the liver with starch and put into boiling water. Then, spinach, spices and salt are added. Eat at one sitting.

d. Bean and date soup. Take mung beans, 50 g, Chinese dates, 50 g, and some brown sugar. Boil the dates and beans until well-cooked. Add the sugar and boil for a few moments more, then administer. This can be taken daily for half to one month.

e. Dried longan pulp and mulberry fruit soup. Boil 15 g of dried longan pulp with 30 g mulberry fruit until the longan pulp swells. Discard the residue, and then add some honey when it has cooled. Take once daily. This may be taken over a fairly long period.

f. Date and auricularia auricula-judae (an edible fungus) soup. Take 30 g of A. auricula-judae, rinse and immerse in water for half an hour. Then boil with Chinese dates (30 pieces) until soft. Brown sugar is then added. Take once daily over a fairly long period of time.

9. Allergic purpura

This ailment is characterized by skin rashes or petechial lesions, coupled with abdominal aches or joint pains.

Prescriptions:

a. Peanut skin soup. Boil 30 g peanut skins with 20-30 g Chinese dates at a low heat until the dates are well done. Throw away the residue and drink the soup. Take once daily for 5-7 days.

b. Chinese dates. Take 10 dates thrice daily for 1-2 weeks. They can also be prepared as a date drink. Take 250 g of Chinese date. Add 1,500 ml water and boil until the dates are swollen. Discard the stones and boil for another 40 minutes. Filtrate, add 300 ml more water to the residue and boil again for another 40 minutes. Filter again and discard the residue. Mix the two filtrates and concentrate it over a low heat to about 750 ml. Drink 250 ml, thrice daily. Effective when administered over a long period.

c. Date and barley soup. Add 500 ml water to 500 g barley and 15 g Chinese dates. Boil at a low heat down to 150 ml and drink it all. Once daily for 1-2 weeks.

d. Thick soup of Chinese date and pig's skin. Take 500 g of pig's skin with all the hairs pulled out and rinse thoroughly. Add an appropriate amount of water and boil at a low heat to make a sticky soup. Then, add 250 g Chinese dates and continue to cook until the dates are well done. Add an adequate amount of sugar, white or brown. Eat at meals, as a side dish, as you like, for any length of time. Also good for hemophilia.

e. Porridge of Chinese dates and Herba Lithospermum: Boil 10 g Herba Lithospermum and 3 pieces of Chinese dates for a while. Discard the residue. Boil 50 g millet in the filtrate with slow fire to make porridge. Take it after cool down. This recipe can be served for a long period.

10. Hypertension

Refers to primary or idiopathic hypertension, rather than hypertension secondary to other disorders, such as nephritis, pheochromocytoma, etc.

a. Jellyfish and water chestnut soup. Desalt 125 g jellyfish by soaking it in water for a whole day. Slice it and 375 g of water chestnuts (with peel) into small pieces. Put them into 1,000 ml of water and simmer over a low heat until 3/4 of the water has evaporated. Filter and discard the residue. Drink the filtrate, 125 ml per dose, twice a day. It can be administered over a long period, and is good for lowering and stabilizing blood pressure.

b. Celery. Celery has a blood pressure lowering action and can be administered in many ways. Cut celery into small pieces and squeeze out the juice. Add sugar, either white or brown, and sip it as one would tea. Celery can also be prepared as a decoction or cooked with balsam pear and eaten as a side dish at meals.

Clinical report: It was reported that celery yields good results on primary hypertension. A group of 16 cases was treated with fresh celery juice together with equal amount of bee honey or syrup, 40 ml. Blood pressure began to decrease on the second day of administration, with better sleep and increased urine. Fourteen cases were effective, with only 2 cases unsatisfactory.

c. Honey. It also has a certain blood pressure lowering action and is effective at the early stage of hypertension. Dilute honey with water and sip it like tea.

d. Mung beans and kelp porridge. Take kelp and mung beans, each 100 g. Boil the mung beans first until they "bloom." Add rice and kelp and simmer at a low heat until sticky. Best eaten in the evenings, it can be taken over a long period.

e. Garlic and mung bean soup. Take 100 g mung beans and garlic, one clove for each year until 50 cloves are reached for those older than 50 years of age. Peel the garlic cloves and put them, with the mung beans, into a bowl. Add 500 ml. of boiling water, cover, and leave to infuse for 10 minutes. Sugar may be added to taste, then drink it like tea.

f. Take a fresh pig's gallbladder, fill it with several cleaned mung beans, then hang it out to dry. When completely dry remove the beans. Take 6-7 beans with water twice a day. Can be administered for a fairly long period.

g. Sea cucumber with crystal sugar. Rinse 30 g sea cucumber and discard its internal viscera. Add crystal sugar and water and simmer at a low heat. Best taken before the midday meal, the whole dose once per day. This can be taken for a long course.

h. Water chestnut and turnip juice. Cut water chestnuts and turnips into pieces, 750 g of each. Wrap in gauze and press out the juice. Add some honey and then bottle. Drink 1 cup of the juice 2-3 times daily. Make fresh juice everyday.

i. Fish head and elevated gastrodia soup. Take a silver carp's head. After rinsing, put it in an earthenware pot with 12 g elevated gastrodia, some Chinese onion, vinegar, water and salt. Cook for more than half an hour. Eat the fish head and soup. This can be eaten regularly.

11. Diabetes mellitus

Dietotherapy is a treatment of decisive significance in diabetes mellitus, which can be effectively controlled provided rational dietotherapy is provided.

a. Sweet potato leaves. Also called white potato or red potato leaves. Take 60 g fresh leaves (30 g dry leaves) and 100 g fresh white gourd's skin (or 12 g dry skin). Cut both into small pieces and boil. Drink in the same way as tea, for any length of time.

b. Chinese yam soup. Take 100 g fresh Chinese yam (or 20 g dried yam) and 20 g Chinese trichosanthes and boil. Drink a bowl of this soup daily for any length of time. This soup may be also prepared by adding a pig's pancreas to 200 g fresh Chinese yam, then boiling with a little salt. Administer once daily, dividing it into 4 doses.

c. Dark plum drink. Infuse 15 g dark plum in boiling water, then drink it like tea.

d. Cowpea soup. Boil 50 g cowpea plus pods for 20 minutes. Drink the soup and eat the peas. Administer once daily.

e. Mare's milk. Drink 125 ml boiled mare's milk twice daily for any length of time.

f. Superior Chinese yam. Steam and peel 500 g Chinese yam. Mix in a bowl with 150 g flour to make a paste. Make small cakes from the paste, garnishing with nuts and preserved fruits. Steam the cakes for 20 minutes. Finally, coat with honey solution (the solution is prepared by mixing one spoonful of honey with 100 g white sugar and some pork fat and starch, then cooking well). One batch of cakes may last 2-3 days.

g. Pig's stomach porridge. Boil a pig's stomach of about 500 g until it is more than half done, and then cut it into slivers. Take rice and the slivered pig's stomach, 100 g each, and cook in the original soup. Add Chinese onion, ginger and garlic before serving.

h. Braised gluten. Fry 250 g gluten for a while and then add ginger and Chinese onion. Add one bowl of water and some salt. When well cooked, add starch solution and continue to cook until it becomes sticky, then serve.

Remarks: In traditional Chinese medicine, it is claimed that the mechanism of diabetes mellitus is chronic depletion of one's body fluid, resulting in *yin*-deficiency and endogenous dry-heat. Hence, the principle for therapy of diabetes is nourishing the *yin*-principle with tonics of moistening nature so that no further aggravation of body fluid occurs. Based on this idea, diabetic victims can maintain their health, leading a normal life even without relying on anti-diabetic remedies. One of my colleagues has been suffering diabetes mellitus for several years. He is in his early sixties. His urine glucose was always strongly positive. However, he followed the dietotherapeutic principle by taking Chinese yam daily as a routine, avoiding all diets of hot, warm and dry nature, including those foods such as fried or baked, and spices, dog meat, goose meat, pepper, and even longan and lichee and the likes. Whenever he felt hungry, he used to take soybean and its products, vegetables, gourds etc. By doing so, he now leads a normal life without much adverse sufferings.

12. Simple goiter

This is an endemic disease due to deficiency of iodine intake. Females are more susceptible, especially in puberty, gestation and lactation stages. It is known that extra consumption of some vegetables, such as cabbage, turnips, walnuts, maize, bamboo shoots, shallot and garlic (in which some unknown ingredients exist), can also cause such disease.

a. Kelp powder. Bake kelp and seaweed, 500 g each, until dry. Grind into powder and take 10 g daily. 250 g may also be made into soup. Take daily for half a month.

b. Laver. May be prepared in many ways; for instance, as a soup, or stir-fried with other ingredients. About 10 g is enough per dose.

c. Oyster and kelp soup: Boil 100 g oyster, 25 g kelp and 15 g Nostoc Commune var. flagelliforme together. Serve it twice a day.

Remarks: It is known that there are also simple goiters due to hyperiodine intake. In some places, such as coastal areas, islands and some isolated areas where the water contains very high iodine concentration (e.g., in Huanghua County of Hebei Province, China), the water from deep wells contains 500-1000 ug/1, 10-20 times more than needed daily. For such cases, the above iodine rich recipes are contraindicated.

13. Nephritic edema

The causes of edema are varied. It may be caused by cardiac, nephritic hepatic, endocrine or nutritional diseases. Therefore, correct diagnosis is imperative before dietotherapy starts.

a. Pig's stomach and lotus seed soup. Thoroughly rinse a pig's stomach and stuff it with 40-50 lotus seeds with their sprouts removed. Sew up the stomach and then boil until well done. Add a little salt and monosodium glutamate. Serve in 2-3 doses. It may also be served in sliver form with lotus seeds. Sesame oil, Chinese onion and garlic may also be added.

b. Cogon root and red bean porridge. Rinse and boil 200 g fresh cogon root (50 g if dried) for half an hour. Discard the residue, then add 50 g red beans and continue to simmer until the beans "bloom." Add 200 g rice and cook until porridge becomes sticky. Take the porridge in 2-3 doses.

c. Calabash soup. Take 50 g calabash with its pulp and seeds discarded, rind of watermelon and white gourd, 30 g each, Chinese dates, 10 g. Add 500 ml water and boil at a low heat until 150 ml is left. Discard the residue and drink the soup once daily. Also good for preventing heat stroke.

d. Take a snake head fish of about 500 g and 50 g of red beans. Clean and gut fish with scales remaining, stuffing its stomach with the beans. Wrap the fish in several layers of thick paper. Stick a piece of lead wire through the mouth of the fish, wind it around the body, then immerse it in fresh water. When the paper is soaked through, embed the fish in a charcoal fire until it is well done. Take it without salt in two doses, for seven successive days as a course.

e. Poria porridge. Pulverize poria into powder and use 15-20 g with a reasonable amount of rice to make a porridge. This can be eaten daily over a long period.

f. Porridge made from membranaceus astragali. Boil 30-60 g fresh astragali at a low heat in 200 ml water until 100 ml remains. Add 100 g rice and some brown sugar and simmer until the rice is well done. Finally add a little tangerine peel powder, bring back to the boil, then it is ready. This porridge can be eaten in the morning or evening, though it is not suitable for those who are deficient, have a fine and quick pulse, and a red tongue.

g. Pig's liver and mung bean porridge. Make a porridge out of 50 g mung beans and 100 g rice. Add 100 g cleaned and chopped pig's liver. Boil the porridge for a little while until the liver is done. There is no need to add salt. This porridge can be eaten regularly.

Remarks: Two cases of edema were treated at a TCM clinic. The doctor, a veteran physician with no biomedicine education recommended the same dietotherapeutic recipes of Poria porridge and snake head fish to be administered alternately for several months. Upon follow-up visit, one of the cases ameliorated remarkably without any visible edema, while the other case complained that the prescriptions had been used to little avail. Reexamination of laboratory indices taken in a hospital of Western medicine revealed that the former was a nephritic patient, while the latter, a cardiac case.

14. Rheumatism of joints and cartilage

In traditional Chinese medicine, rheumatism of joints and cartilage falls under the category of "Bi" syndrome, which is further divided into 3 types on the basis of pathogenic predominance, i.e., cold-pathogen, damp-pathogen and wind-pathogen. The manifestations vary according to which type of pathogen is predominant. For cold type, pain is quite severe; for damp type, pain always stays at a fixed location; and for the wind type, pain is wandering in nature. There are also types of mixed pathogens. The dietotherapeutic recipes should also vary accordingly.

a. Aconite porridge: This is for rheumatic arthritis of cold-type or cold-damp type. Put 50 g rice and 10 g raw aconite powder together in a pot to which 500 ml of water is added. After boiling, simmer with slow fire for a while. Add 1 tea-spoonful of ginger juice, 3 tea-spoonfuls of honey. Continue simmering until rice is well-done. Take it with empty stomach. If 6 g of Job's-tear is added, the effect will be even better.

b. Steamed mutton with monkshood slices is also used for the same type as "a" above: Cut cooked mutton into cubes of 2.5 cm. Put in a large bowl with rinsed monkshood slices. Add millet wine, cooked pig's fat, shallot segments, ginger slices, and broth. Steam it in water bath for 3 hours. Put some small shallot pieces, monosodium glutamate, and pepper powder, and serve as a side dish.

c. Papaya and Job's-tear porridge. For damp-pathogen rheumatism. Rinse 10 g papaya and 3 g Job's-tear. Put them in a small pot and pour in cool water. Immerse for a while and then cook with slow fire until Job's-tear is softened. Add a teaspoonful of sugar and cook again for a while. Take it at anytime. This may be administered on a daily basis.

d. Slender acanthopanax root bark liquor. Soak 50 g acanthopanax root bark in water and then boil at low heat. Pour off the decoction at half and one hour intervals (adding more water after the first time). Take 500 g glutinous rice. After rinsing, add water and boil with the above acanthopanax decoction to make sticky rice. When cold, add some distiller's yeast and ferment to make rice liquor. Serve it as beverage at meal time.

e. Inkfish liquor. Take 2 dried inkfish with bones and put into 250 ml Chinese yellow wine, then boil at a low heat until well done. Drink the wine and eat the inkfish. The amount of wine drunk should vary according to individual tolerance. Drink once or twice daily for several days. For patients with impaired functions of the heart, kidney and liver, it should be administered with care or contraindicated.

15. Vertigo (Meniere's syndrome)

Causes of vertigo are also diversified. Meniere's syndrome is one of the commonest illness. By TCM, it is claimed that when the *yin* principle or blood is deficient, vertigo ensues.

a. Gingko with Chinese date soup. 25 g of gingko's flesh is pulverized after having been baked dry, then kept in a bottle. Boil 50 g of Chinese dates until 100 ml water remains. Take 5 g gingko powder, swallowed with 30 ml date soup, thrice daily for I week.

b. Oolong tea with chrysanthemum: 10 g chrysanthemum and 3 g oolong tea, infused with boiling water. Serve as one would tea.

c. Pork simmered with selfheal: 50 g pork in thin slices are simmered in water with 20 g selfheal with slow fire. Before well-done, add some soybean sauce, vinegar, and sugar. Serve as a side dish.

d. Thick soup of Gastrodia Elata with pig's brain: Simmer a pig's brain with 10 g Gastrodia Elata with slow fire for 1 hour until it becomes sticky. Discard the residue and add some salt. Take it in several parts within a single day.

Remarks: For vertigo due to high blood pressure, please refer to relevant paragraph in this book. For those due to deficient body, the "c" and "d" recipes are quite satisfactory. A housewife of 50 complained of vertigo for 6 months. She had a bad temperament and was easily excited. Vertigo used to occur after quarreling with her husband. She suffered no hypertension. This thick soup was prescribed for her. After a course of 2 weeks, she improved a lot and she recovered totally after another 2 weeks by taking this diet.

16. Epilepsy

a. White (or black) pepper corns and dried turnip are combined in a 1:2 ratio and ground into powder, then kept for administering. Swallow 2 g with warm water thrice daily. This may be administered for a long period. However, an anti-epileptic drug should be administered at the same time when the seizures occur, while this food is good at consolidating the treatment and can be administered for more than a year.

b. Olive-alum cake: Take 5,000 g of pitted olive and crush in a mortar. Boil at a low heat until sticky. Add some alum powder. By this time the weight should be about 1/5 of the original. Store in a bottle. Dilute with water and drink twice daily, 1 spoonful (15 g) each time. Sugar may be added. A month's period of interruption is needed if a second course is to be begun.

c. Vermicelli with scorpion: Oli-fry 3 pieces of scorpion until it becomes crispy. Cut vermicelli made of bean starch into segments of 30 cm. long and oil-fry it until crispy. Put the fried scorpions on the vermicelli and serve. Take it once daily for 7 successive days. In case further such diets are needed, a 2- or 3-day interruption is needed.

d. Carp with red-bean: A live carp with scales and viscera discarded is cleaned as usual. Crush 50 g red beans, 6 g Amomun Tsao-ko and slice 6 g old tangerine peels, all put into the body cavity of the fish. Insert some salt, shallot, ginger and add chicken broth. Steam it for one hour and serve.

e. Pig's kidney with Radix Angelica and Fructus Lycii: Discard the white tissues of 500 g pig's kidney and its capsule. Rinse it thoroughly. Add the Radix and Fructus, each 10 g. Simmer with water until the kidney is well done. Take out the kidney and cut it into thin slices. Put it on a dish and add appropriate amount of soybean sauce, vinegar, ginger chips, sesame oil and serve cold for 4-5 doses, 1-2 doses daily.

17. Headache

As a symptom, headache may be secondary to many diseases. In TCM, it is differentiated into various types, including exogenous and endogenous. For the former, when the exogenous pathogens and its ensuing ailments are cured, headache subsides spontaneously. For the latter, there are three kinds: Deficient type, phlegmatic dampness and blood stasis types. Deficient type manifests mild, intermittent headache, while the other two (excessive) types reveal severe and persistent headache, which sometimes may deviate to one side as migraine.

a. Thick soup of elevated gastrodia tuber with pig's brain. 10 g of elevated gastrodia tuber is boiled with a whole pig's brain for 1 hour at a low heat. Discard the herbal residue and eat the brain and soup at one draught or divide into doses. This soup can be administered often and is good for migraine and nervous headaches.

b. Feather cockscomb seed drink. Soak 300 g feather cockscomb seeds in water and then boil at a low heat. Drain off the water after 20 minutes and then add more water. Repeat this process twice more. Mix the three solutions and concentrate by simmering until it becomes sticky. When cooled, add 400 g white sugar, mix thoroughly and dry in the sun. Then pulverize it into powder and keep in a bottle. Administer in 10 g doses dissolved in hot water, thrice daily.

c. Fish head with Gastrodia Elata: Slice Rhizoma Ligusticum Chuanxiong and poria, each 10 g, and put together with 25 g Gastrodia Elata into water in which rice has been washed for 4-6 hours. Take out the Gastrodia and steam it with rice. Then cut it into slices which are then put into the abdomen of a live carp with scales and viscera discarded. Add some shallot and ginger segments and then steam it for half an hour. This finishes the process and the fish is then served as a side dish.

d. Porridge of Chinese wolfberry fruit, chrysanthemum and glutinous rehmannia: This is for those headaches due to blood deficiency. Cook 15-30 g processed glutinous rehmanniae, 20-30 g wolfberry fruit with water to obtain concentrated solution. Divide it into 2 parts, each mixed with 100 g rice cooked as porridge. Infuse chrysanthemum with boiling water separately and mix it with the porridge just before it is well done. Before finishing cooking, put some rock sugar into the porridge and serve when the rocks dissolve completely.

e. Porridge of Chinese yam and pinellia tuber: This is suitable for headache of excessive type due to profuse phlegm. Boil 30 g pinellis tuber in 800 ml water to obtain a volume of 500 ml. Discard the residue and then put in 30 g powdered yam. Further boil and mix it with some sugar and serve.

18. Diarrhoea

Diarrhoea is a common symptom. In biomedicine, there is a great variety of causes, the commonest ones include acute gastro-enteritis, amebic or bacillary dysentery, parasitosis, or tuberculous enteritis or tumors. The dietetic recipes below are indicated only when these special ailments are excluded.

a. Pomegranate skin and honey paste. Cut 1,000 g fresh pomegranate skin (half weight if dried) into small pieces and boil in water at a low heat. Drain off the liquid at one hour and a half intervals adding more water as required. Mix the 2 solutions and concentrate by simmering until sticky. Add 300 g honey. Once it has returned to the boil remove from the heat and let it cool. Take a spoonful of soup in hot water two or three times a day.

b. Lotus seed cake. Take 50 g lotus seeds with sprouts discarded. Boil at a low heat until soft, then pound into a paste. Cook some rice, either regular or glutinous, and mix it with the paste. When thoroughly mixed, add white sugar, then administer.

c. Pig's kidney thick soup. Take a pair of cleaned pig's kidneys and cut into small pieces after cutting away the white tissue of each piece. Add 12 g rhizoma drynariae and some water. Cook for 1 hour at low heat, then add some salt and flavouring. Take in one draught or 2 doses. This diet may be taken for 1-2 weeks, and is effective for chronic, prolonged and diarrhoea before dawn.

d. Lichee porridge. Crush 50 g dry lichee pulp with 16 g each lotus seeds and Chinese yam in a small mortar. Add water and cook until well done. Rinse 200 g rice, add the above crushed ingredients and sufficient water and cook until the rice is well done. Administer each evening. This is good for diarrhoea before dawn.

e. Gorgon fruit powder. Pulverize 50 g peeled gorgon fruit. Rinse 100 g rice, add the powder and sufficient water and cook until the rice becomes sticky. Good for chronic diarrhoea.

f. Poria cake: Mix together 500 g fine poria powder, 500 g rice powder and 100 g sugar. Make paste with water and make very thin cake by baking on a pan which can be served daily at will.

Remarks: I myself had been suffering chronic diarrhoea for two years in my forties. I received all kinds of biomedical examinations. Unfortunately, no definite and obvious etiology was diagnosed. The diagnosis from several hospitals used to be suspicious of "tuber culosis of intestine," "allergic colitis." Even "tumuors" were ruled out. Luckily, one of my colleagues is an expert specializing in gasteroenlerology (TCM) and I was diagnosed as deficient gastric functions, hyposplenic function in TCM context. Prescription was to take Poria Cake for a long period. Since then, I used to take it daily. After a half-year administration, my chronic diarrhoea subsided gradually and was eventually cured.

19. Allergic asthma

Allergic asthma is differentiated in TCM into four types, i.e., heat, cold, deficient and excessive, and, accordingly, should be treated dietotherapeutically with respective recipes.

a. Egg and turnip. Around the winter solstice, take a turnip (red skin with white flesh) and cut into two equal pieces. Cut a small hole in each half in such a way that when the halves are put together, an egg may be placed in the hole with the rounded end facing upward. Then put a whole egg inside and bind the turnip together with string. Plant the turnip in a flowerpot. Give attention to water, sunlight and temperature to ensure its growth. Eighty-one days after the winter solstice, take the egg out carefully. It shouldn't be rotten, although the yolk may be scattered through the egg white. Cut the turnip into slices, cook for a while and then add the egg and cook for a little longer. No salt should be added. Divide into two doses, taken in one day. Several doses should be prepared at a time, in case any of the eggs goes rotten and should not be used. This recipe may be given for all types of allergic asthma.

b. Gingko. Cook 12 g gingko flesh in water for 20 minutes. Then add honey or white sugar and drink. Administer once daily. Interrupt after one week's dosage. Not suitable for children. It is indicated for excessive and heat asthma.

c. Ginseng and spinach dumpling: Make 1,500 g spinach paste with its leaves. Squeeze out the juice and discard the residue. Slice 10 g ginseng into thin pieces after moistening and then bake it dry. Ground the ginseng pieces as powder. Then mix the spinach paste, ginseng powder together with suitable amount of salt, soybean sauce, Chinese prickly ash powder, and fine pieces of ginger and shallot, and sesame oil. The paste is served as stuffed material for dumplings. This recipe can be served constantly and is indicated for deficient type of allergic asthma.

d. Pork with caterpillar fungus: Cut 150 g pork into pieces and boil it in water for a little while. Put it in a pot and add 10 g caterpillar fungus with other flavouring materials. After boiling, simmer it with slow fire to form concentrated broth. Take it at a draught. It is also good for deficient type.

e. Ephedrine and apricot-nut porridge: Boil 5 g ephedrine herb in 300 ml water for five minutes and discard the herb. Put 15 g peeled sweet apricot nut and boil until almost well-done. Put rice into the solution to make porridge. It is indicated for excessive type allergic asthma.

f. Pig's lung soup with turnip and water chestnut: Cut 150 g white turnip into pieces and slice water chestnut and pig's lung. Cook these three ingredients together until the lung is well done, and serve. It is indicated for heat type.

g. Pig's lung soup of turnip and apricot nut: The process of cooking is the same as in "f", only substitute water chestnut with sweet peeled apricot nut. It is indicated for cold type asthma.

20. Intestinal obstruction due to ascariasis

This ailment mostly occurs in children. For frequent discharging of worms in faeces, severe abdominal pain, vomiting with ascaris or even fecal material, the following dietotherapy is recommended.

a. Sesame oil (peanut oil or rapeseed oil may be substituted). Add the juice squeezed out of 50 g white portion of Chinese onion to 500 ml oil. For children under 15, administer 20 ml every 6 hours, three times in all. For adults, double the dosage.

b. Peanut oil. Boil the oil. After it has cooled, drink a cupful (100 ml.), three successive doses at six hour intervals. Half doses for children.

Note: After the abdominal pains have disappeared, an anthelmintic should be administered.

21. Alcoholic poisoning

a. 15 g tea infused in boiling water for 10 minutes. Drink a large cupful.

b. Put 15 g white sugar in 30 ml vinegar. Dilute with hot water, and when the sugar has completely dissolved, drink.

c. Take 60 g black soya beans. Add a suitable amount of water and heat until boiling, then drink.

22. White hair

Refers to white hair in youngsters. However, it is also good for delaying the appearance of white hair in the elderly.

a. Multiflower knotweed tuber porridge. 30 g of this tuber is boiled in an earthenware pot until a concentrated solution is left. Meanwhile, 100 g rice is cooked and several dates and some rock candy added. Pour in the tuber solution and continue to cook until it becomes sticky. Eat every morning and evening. Do not use iron pots. Contraindicated for chronic diarrhoea.

b. Chinese wolfberry seed porridge. Cook 100 g rice and 30 g this seed until sticky. Take twice a day, morning and evening, and can be taken over a long period.

c. Honey paste for blackening hair. Ingredients include processed multiflower knotweed tuber, 200 g; poria, 200 g; angelica sinensis, 10 g; Chinese wolfberry seed, 50 g; Chinese dodder seed, 50 g; bidentate achyranthes root, 50 g; fructus psoraleae, 50 g; and black sesame, 50 g. Soak all the ingredients in water for one hour and a half, and then boil. Pour out the solution three times, once every 20 minutes, adding more water each time. Mix these three portions and boil at a low heat until it becomes gelatinous. Add an equal amount of honey. Stir thoroughly and boil. Then let it cool down for use. Take one teaspoonful twice daily, morning and evening.

d. Black sesame porridge. Grind 25 g black sesame. Cook with 150-200 g rice to make porridge. This can be taken for a long period.

23. Insomnia

Insomnia patients shouldn't take sleeping pills for a long time so as to prevent drug tolerance or dependance. The advantage of dietotherapy for insomnia is that it can be used persistently without side effects.

a. Wild jujube seed porridge. 30-45 g wild jujube seed, either raw or cooked, is crushed and boiled to make a thick soup. Cook 100 g rice, adding the soup when the rice is half done, then boil until well done. This porridge can be administered for a long course.

b. Mulberry fruit honey paste. Rinse 1 kg fresh mulberry (a half dose if dried) and boil in water. Pour out the solution after 30 minutes. Add more water and boil for another 30 minutes. Pour out the solution, to which the first solution is then added. Simmer this mixture until it becomes sticky, then add 300 g honey and bring back to the boil. Let it cool and store in a bottle for use. Take a teaspoonful, twice daily. The fruit may also be directly boiled with honey at a low heat to make a preserved fruit.

c. Pig's kidney with angelica root, codonopsis pilosula root, and Chinese yam. Clean 500 g pig's kidney by cutting away the white tissues. Put it in a container and add 10 g each of angelica root, codonopsis pilosula root and yam. Add some water and cook until kidney is well done. Take out the kidney and cut into small pieces, cutting rhomic check on the surface. Add flavouring, ginger, garlic and sesame oil and take it in a draught.

d. Longan and jujube seed drink: Boil longan pulp, jujube seeds, each 10 g and 12 g gorgon fruit together to make a drink, and served as one would tea.

e. Thick soup of bamboo leaves, lotus seed, bark of cortex cinnamon: Boil 50 g fresh bamboo leaves, 20 g lotus seeds with slow fire until the seeds are tender and well done. Grind 2 g bark into powder. Stir thoroughly a hen's egg and pour the boiling solution into the egg. Add the bark powder. It can be served either with sugar or with salt.

24. Dyspepsia

Referring to abdominal distention, belching, and regurgitation after meals.

a. Pig's stomach porridge. Thoroughly rinse a pig's stomach of about 500 g and boil in water until 70-80 percent done. Slice it into threads. Then add to 200 g rice and cook until porridge is well done and sticky with the pig's stomach completely done. Take it in 2 doses. This porridge may be administered for a long period.

b. Preserved hawthorn. 500 g pitted hawthorn is put in a pot and cooked in water until nearly dry. Then add 250 g honey and cook again at a low heat until well done. Store in a pot. Effective for dyspepsia due to overeating of meat, weakened spleen and stomach or diarrhoea. Also good for coronary heart disease.

c. Shredded turnip cake. Cut a turnip into slivers. Stir-fry it with vegetable oil and add minced lean pork with a few drops of sesame oil and some monosodium glutamate. Make thin sheets of dough with flour, then wrap up the turnip mixture in them and bake. Eat the cakes as one likes.

d. Spleen benefitting cakes. Wrap up 6 g dry ginger and 30 g large-headed atractulodes root in gauze and boil with 250 g Chinese dates for about one hour. Discard the gauze and continue to cook until the dates are well done. Discard the stones. Take 15 g ground inner layer of hen's gizzard, to which 500 g flour is added. Bake cakes with these flour sheets. It is good for children's dyspepsia.

e. Sugar preserved kumquat. Take 500 g kumquat and press into flat cakes in a clean container. Discard the pips. Immerse the cakes in 250 g white sugar (dissolved in a little hot water for 24 hours). Then heat slowly until the sugar becomes dry. Add another 250 g white sugar, cover with gauze and wait several days before using.

f. Spiced rice crust. Take 60 g rice crust.* Add cinnamomun cassia bark, fructus amomi, pericarpium zanthoxyli, fennel fruit and Rhizoma atractylodis, each 6 g, and grind into powder. Store the powder in a bottle. Dosage: 3-6 g, twice a day (only yellow crust can be used, scorched crust is not applicable).

g. Take 500 g rice crust and fry until yellow. Mix with scorched hawthorn, 60 g, Chinese yam, 120 g and fructus amomi, 30 g. Then grind into powder and store in a bottle. Take 10 g per dose, twice daily. White sugar may be added.

25. Impotence

a. Herba cistanchis porridge. Put 15-30 g herba cistanchis into an earthenware pot with water and boil until quite well done. Discard the residue. Make porridge with 100-150 g of rice, 100 g of mutton may also be added. Add some ginger, bring back to the boil, then it's ready for use. Contraindicated in chronic diarrhoea.

b. Fried chives and walnut. Deep fry 50 g of walnut in vegetable oil. Then fry some chives until about 80 percent done. Mix the two ingredients. Add some salt and then serve at a meal.

c. Duck with Chinese caterpillar fungus. A male duck of about 1 kg is cleaned and viscera discarded, then boiled or steamed in an earthenware pot (or aluminium pot), with 10 pieces of Chinese caterpillar fungus, and some ginger, Chinese onion and flavouring added. First boil strongly and then simmer until well done. Add some salt and serve. Repeat every 2-3 days.

d. Sheep's kidney and Chinese wolfberry leaf porridge. Rinse 500 g of Chinese wolfberry leaves and cut into small pieces. Clean a pair of sheep's kidneys as usual and then cut into pieces. Take 200 g of rice to which the above ingredients are added and then cook at a low heat until well done. Add some salt, Chinese onion and ginger pieces. This diet can be taken often.

e. Fry 200 g of balsam pear seeds and then grind into powder. Store in bottle for use.

Dosage: 10 g twice daily for ten days. Swallow with yellow rice wine.

---

* Rice crust is the yellow crust left on the bottom of a pan when rice is slightly overcooked.

f. Fried sparrow: Tear off the feathers and discard the viscera of 3 sparrows. After rinsed and dried, fry it in peanut oil and then serve. The number of sparrows may increase gradually until 10 are prepared for each day.

g. Lily solution with lotus seeds and pigeon's eggs: Cook 2 shelled pigeon's eggs with 20 g lily and 30 g lotus seeds with slow fire until well done. Add sugar and serve, once daily for 10-15 days.

h. Soft-shell turtle with fritillar bulb and wind-weed rhizome:

Discard the shell and inner viscera of a turtle and cut it into pieces. Mix the other two ingredients together, each 15 g in a large bowl.

Add some millet wine and salt and steam for one hour and serve. The recipe can be administered once each day or every 2-3 days for a period of 2 months.

Remarks: Impotence is a rather common condition. All the above recipes are also good for premature ejaculation at the same time. However, when the patient is a deficient *yin*-principle case with flaring fire, manifesting thirst, night sweats, hot palms and soles in the afternoon, with rapid and slender pulses, the recipes with warm or hot ingredients such as dog's meat, animal testes or external genitalia should be avoided and substituted with mild nourishing ingredients, such as caterpillar fungus, lotus seeds, balsam pear seeds. A young cadre, 35 years old, after having recovered from pulmonary tuberculosis, found himself impotent. He was prescribed a recipe of "kidney tonic" including antler, dog's testes and penis. The condition got worse. After three months of therapy, he suspended the treatment and visited our clinic for further treatment. His condition was diagnosed as kidney-deficiency of *yin* type and he was ordered to stop all warm and hot "kidney tonics." He was prescribed the above "h" recipe for 2-3 months. His condition improved steadily and was totally cured later.

26. Hiccups

a. 15-30 g sword beans with pods are boiled in 200 ml of water. Add 3 pieces of ginger. Boil until half the volume remains. Add some brown sugar. Drink the soup in 2-3 doses within one day.

b. Put 3 g clove and 10 g orange peel in water. Boil for half an hour and drink the solution.

c. Rinse 30 g fresh ginger and crush in a mortar, squeezing out the juice, to which 30 ml honey is added. Take 1 teaspoonful, 2-3 times daily.

d. Bake 50-100 g dry whole lichee, including stones and skin. Then grind into powder. Swallow 10 g with water, twice daily.

e. Fry 6 g dried inner layer of hen's gizzard. Grind it with salt into powder. Dosage: 3 g, thrice daily. Swallow with water.

27. Habitual constipation

Referring exclusively to constipation without obvious causes, not including that due to high fever or obstruction by tumor mass, etc.

a. 500 g sweet potato is rinsed and cut into medium pieces, then cooked. Add salt or white sugar before eating. Administer before going to bed every evening for 15 successive days.

b. Cut 100 g white turnip into pieces. Press to obtain juice. Add 50 ml honey. Administer once daily.

c. Stir-fry equal amount of walnuts and sesame seeds and grind into powder. Take 1 teaspoonful (about 20 g) every evening before bedtime. This may be taken with some honey. This recipe is especially indicated for senile constipation due to shortage of body fluid.

d. Cut 1 kg fresh potato into small pieces and press out the juice. Boil this juice until it becomes sticky. Add an equal amount of honey and boil again until it is concentrated like honey itself. Remove from heat and store in bottle when cool. Dosage: 1 teaspoonful; twice daily before meals or before bedtime.

e. Take 250 g Chinese trichosanthes fruit and discard the flesh, then put in an earthenware pot with a suitable amount of water and 100 g white sugar. After boiling at a low heat, stir into paste to be used as filling. Then make a dough out of flour (750 g), yeast and water. Once risen, roll out into cakes and stuff with the filling, then either steam or bake and serve as a staple food.

f. Cut up an onion of about 100 g into slices. Another 100 g each of white turnip and potato are also cut into slices. Stir-fry the above slices and serve at a meal.

g. Black sesame drink with ginseng: Pound 15 g black sesame in a mortar. Decoct 5-10 g ginseng in 200 ml water and then discard the residue. Add the sesame powder and some white sugar. After boiling, the solution is ready to serve.

28. Hoarseness

Referring only to hoarseness due to common cold, rather than severe laryngits and other disorders, such as laryngeal polyps or tumours.

a. Clean and peel a pear and press out the juice. From time to time drink a mouthful of juice, keep it in the mouth, then swallow it drop by drop.

b. Cut up 30 g old, salted and dried leaf mustard. Boil for a short while. Drink the soup, keeping it in the mouth and swallow bit by bit. Take twice or thrice a day.

c. Soak 50 g raw peanuts in cool water for a whole night. Discard the membranes and cook over a low heat in an aluminium pot until soft. Administer once daily.

d. Olive. Rinse some olives and keep one in the mouth, swallowing the saliva. Repeat according to the condition.

e. Take slices of fresh white turnip. Dosage: 5-10 slices, thrice daily.

f. Press the juice from a fresh turnip and some fresh ginger. Mix the juices, keep in the mouth, then swallow drop by drop.

g. Pork broth with olive and Rhizoma Polygonati Odorati: Take 30 g Rhizoma Polygnati Odorati, 60 g fresh olive with kernels, 100-150 g pork, and boil them together with 4 bowls of water by slow fire until half of the water is gone. Add salt and monosodium glutamate and serve.

Remarks: For patients with hoarseness, whatever the cause, all kinds of deep-fried, fried, baked and crisp foods should be avoided. It is better to take soft liquid food. Spicy, chilly foods, as well as bitter-cold, are also forbidden.

29. Enuresis (bed-wetting)

a. A complete set of hen's intestines is thoroughly cleaned and then baked dry. Grind into powder and add some white sugar. Take after dinner with hot water for three successive days.

b. Cake of cock's intestine. Make cock's intestine powder as above. Then mix with 250 g flour and add some water to make a soft dough. Add some vegetable oil and salt, then bake as cakes. Administer every evening, one set of intestines sufficient for two doses.

c. Poria and yam steamed stuffed bun. First steam poria and Chinese yam, each 100 g, and then make a paste. Mix this with 200 g flour and 300 g white sugar to serve as the skin of the bun. Use white sugar, preserved fruits and preserved plum slivers as the stuffing. Make steamed buns and administer for a 1-2 week period.

d. Steamed chicken with root of membranous milk vetch: A hen is routinely treated and put in a container to which 30 g root of membranous vetch, some salt and thin ginger slices are added. Steam it until the chicken is well done. Discard the ginger and root and serve.

e. Pig's heart soup with dangshen, Chinese angelica and Chinese magnoliavine fruit. Cut open a pig's heart. Fill the cavity with 20 g dangshen, 10 g Chinese angelica, 10 g Chinese magnoliavine fruit with a little salt. Cook it to well done and serve with the drugs discarded.

f. Soybean sprout soup: Cook 500 g soybean sprout with strong fire for 20 minutes. Add a little salt and pork's oil, and serve.

30. Sweating

a. Membranaceous milk vetch root porridge. Make a concentrated solution of this vetch by boiling 30-60 g of the raw material in water. Add some brown sugar and 100 g rice and make a porridge. When done, add a little tangerine peel. This porridge can be administered for a long period.

b. Put 250 g pork (preferably abdominal wall portion) in 500 ml rice wine and cook at a low heat until well done. Add some white sugar. Administer once every two or three days.

c. Eight pig's trotters (half dose for children) are rinsed thoroughly and boiled. Once boiling, simmer at a low heat until the soup becomes thick. Take in a draught. Administer once daily for 3 successive days.

d. Measure 125 g of fresh, cleaned loach, then fry in oil until yellowy-red and simmer in 500 ml of water until 150 ml is left. Add ginger slivers and salt. Take in a draught (eating both fish and soup), once daily for 3 days. For children, it may be taken in 2-3 doses.

e. Soak 150 g black soybeans in 500 ml water for a few hours. Take 9 g dried bean skin. Mix 9 g floating wheat (put the wheat in water, use those grains which float on the surface of the water) with the bean skin and cook to make a soup. Take it in a draught. 9 g membranaceous milk vetch root may also be used, in which case the floating wheat should be reduced to 3 g.

f. Make a soup out of the spongy core of maize, and drink. Good for sweating due to deficiency in postpartum women.

g. Take 120-150 g of the crust which remains on the sides of the pot when cooking bean curd. Boil this crust and drink the soup and the residue.

h. Take Chinese dates and black plums, each 10 pieces, and make a decoction. Administer morning and evening, twice daily for 10 days.

i. Make a decoction from 12 g mulberry leaves which have suffered frost. Take the decoction once daily for 10 days.

Remarks: In modern biomedicine, sweating is claimed to be controlled by the sympathetic nervous system. There are intractable sweating cases very difficult to cure. By TCM, they are differentiated into *yin* and *yang* syndromes which can be controlled accordingly with corresponding therapy. Here are 2 example cases: A male engineer of 40 complained of profuse spontaneous sweating for several years, especially in the palms, trunk and forehead. The condition aggravated when he was in a mood of tension. All Western medicines had been applied to no avail. It was suggested he take the "a" recipe for a long period. Later, he moved to another city, affiliated to a new post. About half a year later, he wrote me that his profuse sweating was totally healed. Another young man of 22, an undergraduate, was always strenuously studying for several years on the campus. He had a thin constitution and used to suffer night sweating, thirst and afternoon "fever," though the temperature never reached 38°C when he felt very "hot." He was suspicious of pulmonary tuberculosis, but all exams, including X-rays of the lungs, revealed negative results. Night sweating was so serious that it even made him sleepless. He came to our hospital for help and was advised to take dietetic recipes "e" and "f" alternately for as long as 5 months. He was cured at the end.

One should bear in mind that sweating is a symptom secondary to some diseases. For instances, hyperthyroidism, shock or collapse, tuberculosis of the lung, bone, intestine, etc. Night sweating used to occur in tuberculosis. Whatever the ailments, when the primary disorders for sweating are cured, sweating would stop spontaneously. The above recipes are only indicated for those cases without obvious primary causes.

31. Hyperlipemia (hypercholesterolemia)

The following foods can be made into drinks taken regularly like tea: (1). Rhizome of oriental water plantain, 6-9 g daily; (2). tuber of multiflower knotweed; (3). root of cogon; (4). wild rice stem; (5). Alfalfa; (6). thick root of Chinese wolfberry; (7). water chestnut; (8). hawthorn. Among them, Nos. (2), (3), (6) can be administered in 12 g doses and made into drinks. The others can be eaten as vegetables.

a. Blood lipid-lowering tea: Grind 60 g dry lotus leaves, 10 g raw hawthorn and raw Job's-tear, 15 g peanut leaves, 5 g tangerine leaves, and 60 g tea leaves into fine powder. Serve this powder in the usual way as serving tea.

b. Immortal's porridge: Decoct 30-60 g tubers of multiflower knotweed. Filtrate and discard the residue. Make porridge with 100 g rice in an earthenware pot with 3-5 pieces of Chinese dates. Before finishing cooking, add some brown sugar or rock candy and serve.

32. Gout

This is a disorder due to dysfunction of purine metabolism. Though its manifestations are somewhat similar to rheumatism, the dietotherapy should be carefully formulated to prevent excessive intake of foods with high purine contents, including seafoods, sardines, animal viscera and broth from animal products. Some vegetables, including spinach, cauliflower, celery, hyacinth bean, are also rather rich in purine contents and should not be overly consumed.

a. Walnut cake. Take 100 g flour, and prepare it as paste with water. Add 50 g walnut, 30 g Chinese yam, and some sugar. Bake in a pan with vegetable oil. This can be served as staple food daily.

b. Egg soup with cabbage, tomato and Job's-tear. Two hen's eggs are stirred thoroughly and boiled in water with 100 g cabbage and 50 g tomato. Prior to this, 100 g Job's-tear is prepared tender and then added to the soup. This recipe can be served as a daily routine.

33. Overweight

Overweight and obese people should bear in mind that slimming can't be accomplished in one move. It needs perseverance. Moreover, other measures, including appropriate physical training and avoidance of too many calories, are also essential.

a. Leaves of oriental water plantain: 9-12 g such leaves are put in a cup, infused with boiling water and left to stand for 15 minutes. Drink as a substitute for tea or coffee for a long course.

b. Cut up 250 g celery and put in boiling water for 5 minutes. Once cooled, add some salt, monosodium glutamate and sesame oil. Chille pepper may also be added. This food can be eaten as a side dish everyday for 2-3 months.

c. Take the spongy core of 3-5 maize rods and infuse in boiling water for several minutes. Take as a substitute for tea or coffee, twice daily. This may be administered for several months.

d. Everyday eat non-refined grain, such as maize powder, Chinese sorghum, barley, sweet potato or brown rice, together with vegetables containing more cellulose (celery, horseradish, wild rice stem, bean curd, or other bean products). Eat mango or apple after meals every day. Perseverance (for at least 3 months) is of vital importance.

e. White gourd porridge: Peel 80-100 g white gourd and cut into small pieces. Put in an earthenware pot with 100 g rice to make porridge. Use the porridge as a routine meal for breakfast and dinner.

f. Slimming tea of lotus leaves: Use 5 g fresh lotus leaves, 5 g hawthorn, 3 g raw seeds of Job's-tear for tea infusion. Use it as tea substitute. It is good for slimming as well as for hyperlipidemia.

g. Spicy mutton fried with Chinese onion: Heat 50 g vegetable oil in which a few Chinese prickly ash and chilli are fried until a little bit brown. Put in 200 g mutton chips, 10 g ginger filaments, and 100 g Chinese onion, and stir-fry for a while. Add salt, monosodium glutamate, vinegar, millet wine and stir for another while. Serve as a side dish. This recipe is good for those overweight cases used to have cold limbs and chilliness.

h. Assorted oolong porridge: Rinse 30 g raw Chinese Job's-tear, 100 g white gourd seeds, 20 g red beans, and cook them together in water until beans become tender. Wrap some dry lotus leaves and oolong tea with a gauze and put it into the decoction. Boil for 7-8 more minutes. Discard the gauze and eat the porridge. This recipe is good for slimming and strengthening the digestive function as well.

Dietotherapy should be cooling down the blood heat-evil and invigorating *qi*.

B. External Problems

1. Urticaria (nettle rash)

a. Divide a bundle of Chinese chives into two halves. One half is cooked for eating and the other crushed in a mortar. Then add some salt and apply locally.

b. Cut 50 g dried taro stem into small pieces and boil in water at a low heat for half an hour. Add some crystal sugar and boil for a while. Eat the whole solution with residue once daily for several days.

c. Boil 15 g maize hair for 20 minutes. Discard the residue and add 100 g sweet fermented glutinous rice and bring back to the boil. Add some white sugar and drink.

2. Boils and carbuncles

In traditional Chinese medicine, boils and carbuncle are claimed to be a result of accumulated inner heat, leading to poison formation in the blood. Hence, greasy, fried, and dry foods are to be avoided.

a. Egg's cake with dandelion: Rinse 30 g dandelion and cut into segments 1-2 cm long. Add 2 thoroughly stirred hen's eggs and some salt. Stir-fry the eggs with vegetable oil and serve as a side dish.

b. Green bean and watermelon peel solution: Boil 100 g green beans in 1,500 ml water for 10 minutes. Discard the residue and add 500 g watermelon peel. After several minutes, the solution is ready to serve like tea in cool condition.

c. Pork broth with green bean and balsam pear: Clean 250 g lean pork and 250 g balsam pear. Cut them into slices. Boil 250 g green beans for 30 minutes and add pork and balsam pear. Continue to boil with slow fire. Add some salt and serve as beverage in cool condition.

3. Tuberculous lymphadenitis

Referring to those mild cases without ulceration and other general manifestations, such as fever, emaciation, night sweating, etc.

a. Pound up 500 g taro. Also soak 500 g jellyfish in water for a few hours. Then cut it and 500 g water-chestnut into small pieces and boil them together. Once well done, discard the residue, mix the soup with the taro paste and stir thoroughly. Bake until dry and keep in a bottle. Dosage: 3-6 g, 2-3 times daily, swallow with water.

b. Steam fresh taro until extremely well-done. Add some salt and soy sauce. Eat once every day as one likes. This may be taken for a considerable period.

c. Put 15 g kelp, 15 g seaweed and 50 g dried lichee pulp in a pot with water and some yellow rice wine. Boil at a low heat until quite well done. Take the soup with all its ingredients once daily. It can be applied for a long time.

d. Put 50 g oyster flesh in water and bring to boil. Then add some garlic and salt. Serve at meals or with noodles. May be administered for a long period.

e. Put 7 lichee stones, 15 g kelp and 15 g seaweed in a pot with some water and yellow rice wine, simmer for more than 1 hour. Drink the soup once daily.

f. Rinse 2 duck's eggs, 100 g peeled garlic cloves and cook in water for 10-15 minutes. After the eggs are done, shell and boil them further for another 3-5 minutes. Take the eggs and soup. This recipe can be used frequently.

g. Mutton soup with root of membranous milk vetch: Cook 180 g mutton in boiling water. After boiling for a while, put the mutton into cool water to remove its fishy smell. Then use an earthenware pot to cook the mutton together with 30 g vetch, 20 g dry longan pulp, 30 g Chinese yam. Add some spicy materials and serve the soup and all the ingredients.

4. Hypertrophic prostatic gland

This is a disorder commonly seen in males after middle age. The main manifestations include difficulty in urination or even dribbling of urine.

a. White gourd and Job's-tear solution: Clean 350 g white gourd and cut it into pieces. Wash 50 g Job's-tear and boil it with the former for 20-30 minutes. Add some sugar. Use it as tea.

b. Pizza cake with poria, tomato and pork: Make stuffed materials with 30 g pork, spices including shallot, ginger, and millet wine. Add 100 g fine poria powder and mix well. Use this mixture to make pizza cake by frying in oil. Then cover with sauce made of 20 g tomato sauce with some sugar and salt, and serve.

c. Water chestnut soup with jellyfish: Infuse 50 g jellyfish in water and cut into elongated pieces. Cut 150 g peeled water chestnuts into slices and decoct them together. Drink it like tea.

C. Female Problems

1. Mastitis

a. Squeeze out the juice of an orange. Add a tea-spoonful of yellow rice wine. Mix the two ingredients. Dilute with cool boiled water. Take twice daily, in the morning and evening, using one orange each time.

b. Grind 30 g Chinese trichosenthes to which 100 ml yellow rice wine is added. Steam in a water bath at low heat for 20 minutes. Take warm, 20 ml per dose, twice a day.

c. Take 30-50 g acanthaceous indigo tuber. Simmer in 250 ml water until only 100 ml is left. Add some yellow rice wine and drink in a draught. Also crush a fresh tuber with salt, add some vinegar to make a paste for local application, once daily.

d. A cup of sweet fermented glutinous rice is warmed. Mash some chrysanthemum leaves and press out the juice. Mix the two and drink. Also, mix some fermented glutinous rice with the chrysanthemum pulp and apply locally, twice daily.

e. Grind 50 g of deer antler into fine powder. Take 3 g with yellow rice wine, twice daily.

f. Simmering pig's trotter with Chinese onion: Clean thoroughly 4 pig's trotters and simmer with 50 g Chinese onion segments and some salt. Serve several times after well done.

g. Ginseng and lotus seed decoction: Put ginseng and lotus seeds, each 10 g, in a small pot. Add 30 g rock candy and steam until lotus seeds become tender. Take all at one meal.

2. Premature menstruation

In TCM, premature menstruation is believed to be due to heat evil in the blood, accompanied by deficient *qi*. Hence, the principle for this problem should be clearing evil-heat and invigorating *qi*.

a. Soft-shell turtle soup with fresh rhizome of rehmanniae:

Remove the inner viscera, head and shell of a 300-500 g soft-shell turtle and cut it into pieces. Put in an earthenware pot with 50 g fresh rhizome, which is cut into pieces. Add appropriate volume of water and some flavouring materials, including salt and monosodium glutamate. After well-done, take it in several parts.

b. Chicken with Chinese angelica and root of membranous milk vetch: 250 g chicken flesh is mixed with 30 g vetch and 20 g angelica in an earthenware pot with water. Boil first with strong fire and then simmer with slow fire. After done, add flavouring materials and serve. Apply it thrice a week.

3. Delayed menstruation

The mechanism of this disorder is just the reverse of the preceding and should be treated in an opposite way.

a. Mutton broth with Chinese angelica and fresh ginger: Cut 250 g mutton and cook it in an earthenware pot with 30 g angelica and 10 g fresh ginger with slow fire until mutton is well done. Add some flavouring materials. Take the broth. This is especially good for postpartum women with delayed menstruation.

Remarks: Several years ago, one of my niece gave birth. Though she appeared rather healthy and breast-fed her baby, half a year later her menstrual period appeared irregular. Several months later her periods became delayed, with one period each 40-50 days. The blood appeared pink in colour. She was diagnosed with delayed menstruation and given the above recipe for 3 months, one dose every week. She recovered totally after the dietotherapy.

b. Sesame and brown sugar drink: This is much simpler than the above recipe. Clean 50 g black sesame and dry-fry it. When it is still hot, pour in 20 ml millet wine and add 150 g brown sugar. Take a dose daily for 7 successive days.

c. Beef broth with black bean and Chinese angelica: Fry 30 g black beans for a while. Put it into an earthenware pot. Add 20 g angelica and 100 g sliced beef and cook until done. Add some flavours and serve.

4. Leucorrhoea

Referring to profuse vaginal discharge. The following therapies are not indicated for leucorrhoea due to trichomonads.

a. Pork and inkfish soup. Rinse and treat 2 fresh inkfish of about 300 g and discard their bones and viscera. Cook with 250 g lean pork. Add some salt and flavouring. Take once daily for 5 days.

b. Rinse 250 g fresh lotus root and put in an earthenware pot with about 1 litre of water. Cook until only 7-800 ml is left and drink the soup. Repeat for 7 days as a course. It's good for sticky, yellow leucorrhoea.

c. Baked egg. Take 10 hen's eggs, make a small hole in each, and pour in 10 g white pepper powder. Then enclose the whole egg with dough and bake the eggs on coals until well done. Take one egg daily for 10 days as a course. An interval of 3-5 days should be allowed if a second course is necessary.

d. Cut 50 g fresh Chinese chives into segments of 0.3 cm length. Immerse 30 g dried scallop flesh in yellow rice wine for a while. Cook the scallop with the chives and take once daily.

e. Cook 30-60 g crust from a pot used for cooking bean curd, an egg and 1 sheet of the skin of soybean milk together. Take before breakfast in one draught.

f. Bake dry 10 g gingko flesh in an earthenware pot and then boil with some white sugar. Take the gingko flesh and the soup. One can also grind the flesh into powder and administer. Also, gingko powder may be put into an egg through a small hole in the shell. The hole is then covered with paper and the egg steamed. Take 1-2 eggs each day.

g. Boil 15 g eggplant flowers with 30 g Smilax glabra and drink once daily for a week.

h. Take sunflower stem and cut it and its core into pieces. Place 15-30 g in water and heat until it is just boiling. Take twice daily in the morning and evening.

i. Heat 20-30 g of dry broad bean flower in water until it boils for a while, then drink. Take daily.

j. Take the scales from two crucian carp or carp. Boil the scales at a low heat until it becomes sticky. Take with warmed yellow rice wine once daily for a week.

5. Dysmenorrhea

a. Hawthorn wine. Put 500 g dried pitted hawthorn into a wine bottle. Add about 500 ml Chinese white liquor (contains 60 percent alcohol). Cover tightly. Drink after 1-2 weeks. Take 10 ml twice daily.

b. Put 100 g cleaned saffron in a bottle. Add 400 ml Chinese white liquor (60 percent alcohol). Leave to infuse for one week, shaking the bottle everyday. Take 10 ml each day.

c. Boil together 24 g sliced fresh ginger, 9 g Chinese prickly ash and 10 Chinese dates. Take in two doses every day for 1-2 weeks.

d. A sunflower disc (with seeds removed) of about 30-60 g is cut into small pieces and boiled for a short time. Add 30 g brown sugar. Take two doses every day, in the morning and evening.

e. Analgesic porridge of eliminating blood stasis: Decoct 15 g Bulbus Allii Macrostemi, 20 g root of red rooted salvia, and 20 g peach nut in 200 ml water for 20 minutes. Discard the residue. Add 100 g rice and prepare it as porridge. Add some rock candy before serving.

f. Simmered pig's stomach with prickly ash and monkshood: Clean a pig's stomach thoroughly into which insert 2 g Chinese prickly ash, 2 g monkshood, 30 g rice and some Chinese onion. Tie the stomach with a coarse thread and simmer under slow fire until well done, and serve.

6. Insufficiency of postpartum milk secretion

a. 2-4 pig's trotters are thoroughly cleaned and boiled at a low heat for more than 1 hour until done. Add a little salt and take (including soup) once daily. 9-12 g pangolin scales or rice-paper plant may also be added to the soup during preparation.

b. Stew a fresh live crucian carp of about 120 g together with a pig's trotter until well done. Add some salt. Eat one or two pieces daily for 1-2 weeks.

c. Clean and scale a carp as usual. Add some water and onion segments, ginger shreds and salt. Steam or stew until done and eat (including soup).

d. Fry 250 g black sesame over a low heat. Clean a pig's trotter as usual and stew to make a soup. Take 16 g of the sesame with the soup twice a day. The trotter should also be eaten.

e. Clean 500 g pig's liver and cut it into slices. Add 60 g root of membranous milk vetch. Boil it for 10-15 minutes and serve.

7. Lactation cessation

Lactating women with profuse secretions of milk need dietotherapy when requiring the interruption of breastfeeding.

a. 200 g barley, after rinsing, is covered with gauze and kept in a warm place. After sprouting, take 50 of barley sprouts and boil. Drink 1-2 times daily for 1 week. The sprouts should be about 1-2 cm long.

b. Make wheat sprouts with 200 g of wheat in the same way as above. Fry the wheat sprouts until nearly scorched, then boil to make a soup. Drink daily in 3 doses for several days.

c. Stir-fry 60 g wheat bran until yellow. Add 30 g brown sugar. Mix thoroughly and fry again for a short while. Take several times a day. This recipe provides enough for 2 days.

d. Make a decoction from barley and wheat sprouts, each 60 g. Take in one day, divided into two doses for three successive days.

e. Hawthorn drink: Clean and rinse 20 g hawthorn. Cook it in water until well done. Add some sugar and serve in the amount as one likes.

f. Prickly ash and brown sugar drink: Soak 30 g Chinese prickly ash in

400 ml water for 1 hour. Boil it until half the water volume is gone. Then add 30 g brown sugar and serve at one draught, once daily. 2-3 doses will be effective.

D. Childhood Problems

1. Chicken pox

a. Cut 100 g carrot and 60 g fresh coriander into small pieces and boil for a while. Discard the residue and drink the soup once daily.

b. Put 60 g glycine soja and 60 g red beans in a pot with some water and bring to boil. Drink as a tea substitute, once daily.

2. Eczema

a. Thick soup of maize long hairs and lotus seeds: Boil 10 g maize long hairs. Take out the hairs and then add 50 g lotus seeds and 15 g rock candy into the solution and simmer until the seeds become tender, and serve.

b. Carp soup with red bean: Treat the carp as routine. Boil 30 g red beans to tender and add the routinely treated carp until well done. Then it is ready to serve.

c. Yam and poria pudding: First steam 200 g raw Chinese yam, and pound it as paste after done. Boil 100 g Chinese dates and then discard their stones. Mix thoroughly 100 g fine poria powder with the dates and yam paste. Then steam it as pudding. After done, cover its surface with honey.

3. Anorexia

Children's anorexia is somewhat different from that of adults; in the latter it occurs because of fear of overweight and obesity. Childhood cases may be due to immoderate meals, resulting in severe digestive disturbance. This could be manifested in sallow complexion, emaciation, general malaise, but with intact consciousness and mental state.

a. Hawthorn pudding: Grind 100 g rice with 30 g stoned hawthorn into powder. Mix with water and sugar, and then steam to make pudding. Serve it as you like.

b. Pig's stomach porridge with rhizome of large-headed atractylodes: Rinse the stomach thoroughly (about 500 g). Cut into small pieces. Mix with 30 g rhizome of large-headed atractylodes, 10 g arecanut and some ginger, and boil for 20 minutes. Discard the residue. Prepare porridge with the solution. Add flavourings including Chinese onion, monosodium glutamate and serve. One dose for every 3-5 days. A 3-day interruption is needed when a second dose is to be given.

c. Spleen-benefitting cake: Grind 20 g rhizome large-head atractylode and 10 g dry inner layer of chicken gizzard into powder. Bake it to brown colour. Steam 50 g Chinese dates without stones and then prepare as paste with peels discarded. Grind 6 g dry ginger into powder form. Mix all the above ingredients and prepare as cake 0.4 cm thick, 6 cm in diameter. Bake it to make cakes. This is good for children's anorexia of deficient cold spleen and stomach (digestive) function.

E. Problems of Eyes, Nose and Throat

1. Fishbone in throat

a. Boil 10-20 black plums in an earthenware pot at low heat until a concentrated solution is obtained. Drink a mouthful of solution and swallow it slowly drop by drop. The plum flesh may also be swallowed.

b. Take the gallbladder of a mandarin fish and dry it in the shade. Grind into powder once dry and store in a bottle ready for use. Take 0.1-0.2 g and swallow with yellow rice wine.

c. Take an olive stone. Grind with water in a coarse porcelain pot. Swallow the juice.

Remarks: When all kinds of dietotherapy fail to produce desired effect, one should not hesitate to ask the help of a laryngologist.

2. Epistaxis (nasal bleeding)

Referring to nasal bleeding which occurs without obvious causes and cannot be cured by ordinary methods.

a. White turnip juice. Rinse 500 g white turnip and cut into small pieces. Wrap with gauze and press to obtain juice. Take 50 ml and add white sugar before drinking. Administer thrice daily.

b. Steamed lotus root and rice cake. Take lotus root powder, rice powder and white sugar, each 250 g. Mix with an appropriate amount of water to form a paste and steam. Take as many as one likes, two or three times daily.

3. Sty

a. Yam coated with sugar: Clean and peel 500 g Chinese yam, and cut into rhombic pieces. Soak in boiling water for a little while and let dry. Then fry in oil until half done with a brown crust. Put 50 g vegetable oil in a frying pan and heat to about half boilling. Put 150 g white sugar and heat until bubbles appear. Put the fried yam into pan and take pan away from fire immediately. Stir thoroughly and serve. When a piece of yam is pulled out of the oily-sugar, sugar filaments are formed. Serve once daily for 3-4 days.

b. Soak 50 g white chrysanthemum and 5 g raw glycyrrhiza root, and boil 10 minutes. Discard the residue. Serve it hot like tea.

4. Redeye

In biomedicine, this is called acute conjunctivitis, manifesting red eyes, with swelling, pain and profuse secretion, photophobia.

a. Chrysanthemum tea: Pound 100 g white chrysanthemum and 50 g green tea as coarse powder and equally divided into small bags, each 15 g. Infuse it as tea with 1 bag and use as tea substitute.

b. Cold garlic and cucumber: Take 2 fresh and tender cucumbers. Crush them to pieces. Put 4 smashed cloves of garlic and add some flavourings, including vinegar, sugar, and serve.

c. Fry green peel of watermelon: Peel the green portion of a watermelon. Cut into small segments and fry it in oil. Serve as sidedishes.

5. Running nose

Referring to those cases with running nose irrelevant to common cold or flu. It can be the result of chronic rhinitis, nasal sinusitis, with accompanying decrease or even loss of olfactory function, stuffy nose and headache.

a. Purslane porridge with flower buds of lily magnolia: Decoct 10 g of these flower buds for no more then 10 minutes. Use the decocted solution to make 50 g rice porridge. Before done, add 30 g purslane and boil further for several minutes. Administer as breakfast. This recipe is good for thick and yellow nasal discharge.

b. Balsam pear paste: Use a complete piece of balsam pear and pound it as paste, mix 60 g sugar and let stand for 2 hours. Filter and discard the residues. Drink the filtrate cool. This is good for running nose with thick and yellow discharge.

c. Duck with white gourd: Cook a duck by routine process. Put pieces of peeled white gourd with seeds discarded until the duck is well done and serve.

6. Sore throat

Referring to pain in the throat due to other causes than tonsillitis and laryngitis, mostly occurring in diseases such as acute and chronic pharyngitis.

a. Olive and dark plum solution: Use 60 g olive with stone and 10 g dark plum, all slightly pounded. Add 300 ml water and decoct to 100 ml. Discard the residue and add some white sugar. Take 20 ml, 5 times daily.

b. Shallot white solution: Use two bulbs of Chinese onion with roots intact. Boil 6 g root of balloon flower with 3 g root of glycyrrhiza for 5-7 minutes. Add onion white with roots and simmer for 1-2 more minutes. Drink it hot twice in the morning and evening.

Remarks: Chronic sore throat is closely related to smoking and over consumption of spicy foods. I treated a friend of mine who is a poet and a heavy smoker. He used to work late at night and smoke a lot. He suffered itching throat with mild sore throat, tending to cough a little in the morning. I prescribed the "a" recipe for him with a course of 3 months. Under my advise, he quit smoking gradually over a period of 3 months. Since then, he has completely recovered with no more sore throat nor even any itching. He now enjoys the overtime he puts into his work.

VII. Common Medicinal Foods

As mentioned above, there is no sharp demarcation between medicines and foods. Some foods can be purchased from a drug store, some drugs from a grocery shop. Among these, some may be natural products and some artificial. Here introduced are 100 kinds of medicinal foods which are in common use and easily obtained. The items mentioned include: Its scientific Latin name (if available), nature and flavour, actions, indications, scientific chemical analysis and, last of all, therapeutic action.

A. Plants

1. Chinese onion (shallot)

A herbaceous vegetable belonging to the lily family with many species, including the Chinese onion, onion, shallot, scallion, etc. In general, the white portion (the bulb) is used for medicinal purposes.

Nature and flavour: Pungent, warm, non-toxic.

Constituents: Carotene, vitamins B_1, B_2, and C, calcium, iron, magnesium, volatile oil and allium.

Actions: The volatile ingredients in onion bulb is bacteriostatic to many microbes, including bacilli of diphtheria, tuberculosis, dysentery, streptococcus and staphylococcus. Its water infusion (1:1) also reveals inhibition on pathogenic fungus of the skin in vitro.

Clinical report: Chinese onion is a very common medicinal vegetable. All parts are used. The green part is

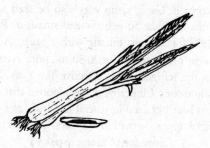

smashed and applied locally for boils and carbuncles or mild trauma. The white bulb is the most commonly used part. Clinically, 107 cases were treated by rubbing onion white paste with equal part of ginger contained in a gauze on body parts including the chest, back, soles, palms, axillae and popliteal fossae. All these cases recovered within 1-2 days. Onion juice may also be used.

2. Garlic

A perennial plant of the lily family. The cloves of its underground bulb are used for medicinal purposes. A bulb with a single clove is preferred.

Nature and flavour: Pungent and warm with stimulating odour.

Constituents: Containing allicin, a volatile oil with stimulating odour. Also vitamins A, B, and C, cellulose, and minerals including calcium, phosphorus and iron.

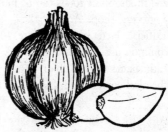

Actions: Allicin, the main ingredient contained in the garlic and the source responsible for its special odour, is bactericidal to pathogenic microbes of dysentery, typhoid and paratyphoid, pneumonia and diphtheria. It also reveals antitussive and expectorating actions. Also good for epidemic meningo-encephalomyelitis.

Recipe examples: For dysentery, take one raw bulb of garlic. Since allicin is heat labile, it is advisable to use it raw. Cooking is not recommended. Use one bulb daily. Excess dosage will be harmful to eyesight and irritable to stomach. Garlic syrup may also be used to protect the stomach from being irritated. Take 50 g garlic and smash it. Put it in 100 ml water and keep at 38°C for 2 hours. Filtrate with a gauze. Add half volume of syrup (made by sugar plus water). Use 20-30 ml, once every 4-6 hours. The syrup, when kept in the refrigerator, is effective for 1 week. Purple peel bulb is better than white ones. Clinically, it was reported that an effective rate of over 95 percent has been obtained in several hundred cases of bacillary dysentery, with normal stool appearing within 2-4 days, on average.

3. Coriander (Chinese parsley)

A mono-rennial vegetable. The whole herb is used for medicinal purposes.

Nature and flavour: Pungent and warm with special fragrance.

Constituents: Volatile oil, fatty acid, decanal, nonahal, and linalool.

Actions: In traditional Chinese thought, the condition of skin rash appearing in measles or German measles is an indication for its prognosis.

Full eruption is believed to have a good prognosis. While those with scarce and gloomy eruptions are susceptible to complications such as pneumonia and other problems. Hence, assistance in skin rash eruptions is one of the best remedies for measles. Coriander is good to use in skin eruptions.

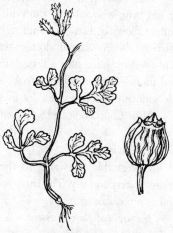

Remarks: Use coriander at the right time, i.e., at the early stage of the disease when skin rash is scarce. When the disease enters its 3rd day or over, when eruptions are very dense, do not use it further, or the condition will be aggravated. Use it as a seasoning with other foods the patient likes. At the same time, decoct it and use the decoction as a wash to eliminate eruptions.

Recipe example: Cut 50 g coriander into small pieces. Fry it with 200 g shredded pork and add suitable amount of soybean sauce and onion pieces. Serve as a sidedish.

4. Chinese chives

A perennial vegetable of the lily family. The whole plant, seeds and root are used for medicinal purposes.

Nature and flavour: Pungent, sweet, warm and nontoxic.

Constituents: Containing volatile oil and sulphurous compounds, carrotene and vitamins B and C.

Actions: Generally, roots off chives are used for activating blood, trauma, difficult swallowing and bleedings, including nasal bleeding, hemoptysis and prolapse of anus. The seeds are good for impotence, frequent urination, seminal emission. Chive root is also good for all kinds of bleeding. The whole plant is also indicated for constipation and gastroenteritis.

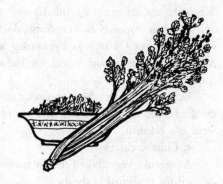

Case example: It is reported that an old man, who suffered from difficult swallowing, used to vomit right after meals. A veteran doctor prescribed chive juice plus a little brine and plum. The remedy was to be swallowed bit by bit, increased gradually. He suddenly vomited out a lot of sticky slivery mucus and was cured.

Note: Contraindicated in patients of deficient vital essence with excessive evil-fire.

5. Celery

A vegetable belonging to the daucas family. There are two kinds of celery, watery and dry. The latter is commonly applied for medicinal purposes and is more aromatic.

Nature and flavour: Sweet and cool.

Constituents: Containing apiin, bergapten, aromatic butylphthalide, volatile oil, carotene. It is also rich in vitamin C and with a large amount of cellulose.

Actions: It is good for hypertension. It also reveals a sedative action, usually applied in menstrual disorders; especially dysmenorrhea.

Clinical report: A group containing 16 cases of primary hypertension was treated by this method. Results indicated 13 cases saw their blood pressure begin to drop by the next day with better sleep and increased urination. Another report mentioned that in the laboratory experiments, decoction from fresh celery leaves yields actions of blood tonic similar to liver extract. In animal experiments, active ingredients from its seed extract also yield bacteriostatic action.

Case example: A male teacher, 40 years old, complained of constant headaches and dizziness, especially in the morning. He was discovered to have moderate high blood pressure of primary type (B.P. 160/100 mmHg). He was advised to have low sodium diets, preferably vegetarian food with celery as his major dish. On this order, the patient basically consumed a vegetarian food regime, without administering any depressor. Upon examination a year later, he was found to have a normal blood pressure, only at its upper margin of 135/90 mmHg.

Remarks: Celery is mostly applied for lowering high blood pressure, as well as high blood cholesterol. In addition to its daily use as a routine food, its depressive action may be obtained by squeezing rooted celery and adding equal amount of bee honey or syrup. Use 40 ml, three times a day.

6. Cogongrass root

A plant belonging to the grass family with a white segmented root rich in water. The juice is sweet.

Nature and flavour: Sweet and cold.

Constituents: Containing coixol, arundoin, cylindrin, glucose and sucrose.

Actions: Animal experiments show that cogon root possesses diuretic action, also with some antibiotic action.

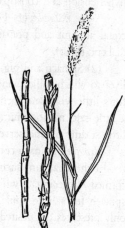

Clinical report: Many reports revealed that cogongrass root is a rather effective remedy for acute nephritis. It was reported that a group of 70 cases of acute nephritis had total daily urine volume of 1,500-3,000 ml 1-5 days after cogongrass administration. Laboratory exams showed normal urine. Blood pressure returned to normal too. It also possesses some antipyretic action. The flower cools the blood with some hemostatic action. It was also reported that 21 cases of acute hepatitis (type A) out of 28 were cured with a daily dose of 100 g of cogongrass decoction. All the symptoms subsided within a period of 45 days. The other 7 cases were markedly ameliorated.

7. Spinach

A vegetable belonging to the chenopodiacea family. The whole plant is used for medicinal purposes.

Nature and flavour: Sweet and cold.

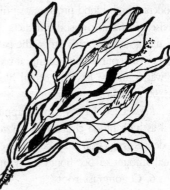

Constituents: Protein, cellulose, carrotene, vitamins B_1 and B_2 and C, oxalic acid, calcium, phosphorus, and high iron content. It also contains some zinc and spinacetin, patuletin in trace amount.

Indications: Since spinach is cold and rich in iron, it is indicated in anemia of iron-deficiency type. It also yields some effect on hypertension and constipation, and is also effective for thirst.

Recipe example: (1) Use spinach root, inner lining of chicken gizzard in equal amount and prepare as powder. Dosage: 3 g three times a day (for diabetic thirst).

(2) Spinach and pig liver soup: Pig liver 150 g; spinach 250 g. Slice the liver to which millet wine and corn starch are added. Boil the slices in water for a little while and then put in a bowl. Put spinach into boiling water. Add a little salt, monosodium glutamate and then pour it into the bowl. Add a little sesame oil and serve.

Remarks: Spinach contains rich oxalic acid. When spinach is cooked with food rich in calcium such as soybean curd, sea foods, calcium oxalate will be formed as precipitate which is unabsorbable. To avoid, it is advisable to boil spinach for a little while and discard the solution before cooking. This not only preserves the desired calcium but also eliminates puckery taste of oxalic acid. Children are advised not to eat too much spinach which may cause diarrhoea. For the same reason, it is also contraindicated in males suffering premature ejaculation.

8. Purslane

A plant belonging to the purslane family. The whole grass is used for medicinal purposes.

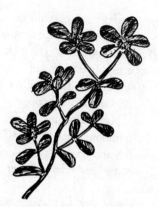

Nature and flavour: Sour and cold.

Constituents: It contains rich noradrenaline and potassium compounds, dopamine, glucose, cellulose, carrotene, calcium, phosphorus, iron and vitamins B_1, B_2 and C.

Experiments: In vitro experiments showed a concentration of 1:4 solution revealing bactericidal action on dysentery bacilli and Eschericher coli. Clinically, it has been reported that fresh purslane porridge yields preventive action on epidemic dysentery in several thousand cases observed. In a comparative study, it was shown that wild fresh purslane yields anti-dysentery action similar to that of sulfonamides and synthomycin.

Recipe example: Prepare 2 large bundles of this wild herb and cut into small pieces. Boil it with rice to make porridge. No salt is to be added.

9. Peppermint

A plant belonging to the labiata family. The *longnau* peppermint produced in Suzhou, China, is especially famous. The whole plant is used for medicinal purposes.

Nature and flavour: Pungent and cool.

Constituents: Volatile oil with menthol, camphene, menthone, limonene.

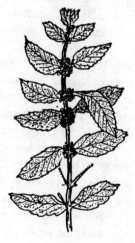

Actions: 77-78 percent of the volatile oil contained in peppermint, which is responsible for the cool perception when applied to body surface, is menthol. Local application of peppermint relieves local pain and itching of warm nature. Some kinds of severe pain may be cured by peppermint, including neuralgia such as trigeminal neuralgia, headache, toothache and sore throat.

Recipe examples: 1. Decoct 10 g fresh peppermint in water and serve as tea drink for sore throat after adding some sugar. Do not use in cold type sore throat, i.e., without redness and rapid pulse, etc.

2. Use 9 g peppermint (for fresh specimen, the dose may increase to 20 g) and cook with 100-150 g bean curd. After boiling for less than 5 minutes, take it hot. It is indicated for common cold of wind-heat type, manifesting stuffy nose, mild fever with a little sweating.

10. Capillary artemisia

A plant belonging to the composita family. Its young sprout is served as a common vegetable in China. It is collected in the 5th month (lunar calendar) and used as a medicine.

Nature and flavour: Bitter and slightly cold.

Constituents: Containing scoparon, caffeic acid, capillone, capillene, capillarine, fatty acid and potassium chloride.

Action: In animal experiments, it reveals cholagogic action, lowering blood pressure, diuretic and anti-microbial actions.

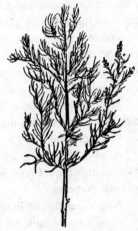

It also possesses antipyretic and expelling dampness in the body. Commonly applied in infectious hepatitis (jaundice type), cholecystitis and measles. Also used as a subsidiary treatment in hypertension, nephritis and liver cirrhosis.

Clinical report: Capillary artemisia has long been used as a cholagogic remedy for treating jaundice in China. It was reported that 32 cases of acute viral hepatitis A were treated with capillary artemisia (50-75 g decocted and taken 3 times a day). The course of treatment averaged 7 days, with jaundice and fever subsiding rapidly. No side effects and relapse were observed.

Recipe example: Use 100 g artemisia and fry with 50 g pork slices for 2 minutes. Then add some salt, monosodium glutamate and serve as a side dish. It is good for convalescent stage of hepatitis patient and can be served daily.

11. Auricular auricular-jade (an edible fungus)

This is a kind of fungus parasitic on the surface of woody and decayed trees where the weather is damp. It belongs to auriculariae family and appears in the form of a human external auricle.

Nature and flavour: Sweet, moderate, and glossy.

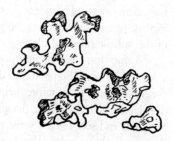

Constituents: It is rich in protein. Each 100 g contains 10.6 g protein, 357 mg calcium, 201 mg phosphorus, 185 mg iron. It also contains carrotene, vitamins B_1 and B_2, mannan, glucuronic acid, lecithin, and cephalin.

Action: It is a very good blood tonic, containing 7 times as much iron as pig's liver. It also possesses powerful inhibitions to the agglutinating tendency of blood platelets and helps to lower the level of blood lipids, including blood cholesterol. Recent reports reveal that constant consumption of this fungus is also helpful for the prevention of tumours.

Remarks: There are two kinds of this edible fungus, black and white. Formerly, the black fungus was a common food in daily use, while the white was claimed to be a good tonic. Nowadays, both fungi can be cultivated in the garden and the white fungus is also commonly applied.

Recipe examples: (1) For sore throat and coughing. Take 15 g white fungus. Immerse in boiled cold water for an hour. Filtrate and discard the water. Steam with water and rock candy with slow fire for 2-3 hours until sticky. Use once a day. It is good for the infirm with constant coughing, deficient *yin*, manifesting low afternoon fever, thirst, headache and general malaise.

(2) For anemia. Immerse 15 g black fungus and 15 pieces of Chinese red dates in water for 1 hour. Add some rock candy and steam with slow fire for another hour until sticky. Serve twice daily.

(3) For anemia and the infirm. Use 15 g dry black fungus, 4 hen's eggs, 100 g spinach, 100 g pork in slices of shreds. Fry each ingredient separately and then mix together to serve as a side dish.

12. Cinnamon bark

A plant belonging to the lauracea family. It is a common seasoning meteria in Chinese way of cooking. The barks are collected in winter and dried in the dark. Sometimes its leaves may be used as a flavouring substance.

Constituents: One percent of the bark is volatile oil in which the common ingredients are phellandene, eugenal, methyleugenol. In the leaves, 60 percent of the volatile oil is safrole.

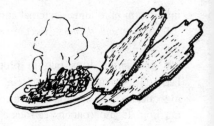

Action: It is warm and good for stomachache of cold type. It also dredges the vessels and is therefore helpful to dispel cold and rheumatic disorders of the joints and soft tissues, waist pain of damp and cold type. It is also good for menstrual pain, postpartum symptoms with body pains of cold type.

Recipe example: Use 10 g cinnamon bark to cook with 150 g pork under low fire until the pork is well done. Eat the pork and drink the soup. It is a common recipe for rheumatism. However, cases of deficient *yin* type is contraindicated due to the warm and pungent nature of the bark.

13. Tea

A perennial plant belonging to the camellia family. One of the most popular beverages in the world.

Nature and flavour: Sweet, bitter and slightly cold.

Constituents: Very complicated. Mainly containing caffeine, theophyline, cocaine, tannate, theobromine, geranial, vitamins B_1, B_2 and C, ergosteroid, volatile oil, theaspirone, etc.

Experimental results: It was reported that tea reveals both anti-senility and anti-tumour effects. It regulates and delays the process and advent of senile and physiological changes in the organism. Reports showed that the extracts from tea greatly decrease rate of mortality of the duplet lung cells of human embryo than the control group. Tea, especially red tea, prolongs the life of drosophila flies in the lab. It also lowers the level of blood lipids and effectively prevents the development of hypertension, coronary disease and arteriosclerosis. Tea is also a good antidote and delays the absorption of toxic substances such as alkaloid and metallic salts.

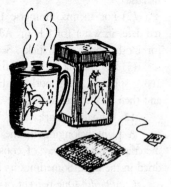

Clinical report: For dysentery: Decoct

10 g tea for 10 minutes and then add a few drops of sesame oil. Clinical reports claimed that up to several hundred cases of acute and chronic dysentery, when treated with 100 percent tea decoction administered 2-10 ml 3-4 times a day, revealed a cured rate of 95 percent and 85 percent, respectively. It is also claimed that investigations show that drinking tea as daily beverage results in a lower incidence of coronary heart disease and lower blood cholesterol level.

Remarks: It is advisable that in order to preserve as much vitamin C as possible, one should not use 100°C boiling water to make tea for drinking. Instead, boiled water at 60-70°C is preferable.

14. Seaweed

Belonging to the sagossum family.

Nature and flavour: Salty and cold.

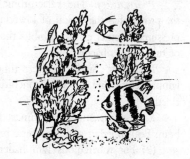

Constituents: Sargassum fusiforame contains alginic acid, protein, mannitol, potassium and iodine. Sargassum pallidam contains alginic acid, protein, mannitol, potassium and iodine. Besides, it also contains sargassan, etc.

Actions: In animal experiments, it reveals anti-coagulant action, lowering of blood fat and blood pressure. It also demonstrates temporary restraining of the rise of metabolic rate due to hyperthyroidism and is applied in the preparatory stage before thyroid operations. It also reveals inhibitory action on some tumours (Erlich ascites cancer and uterine cancer).

Experimental report: It yields an action which inhibits hyperthyroid secretion similar to that of kelp. Alginic acid possesses an action to prevent hypofunction of blood coagulation. Hence, it can be used for patients with a tendency to hemorrhage.

Recipe examples: (1) For simple goitre. Boil 50 g seaweed, after thoroughly rinsed, under slow fire until half of the original water volume is evaporated. Drink once a day for several months.

(2) For lumps such as swelling lymph glands or testes. Use seaweed and kelp, each 20 g, caroway seeds 5 g. Boil together in water under slow fire

and drink daily for a considerable period of 3-4 months.

(3) For chronic bronchitis. Cut 100 g seaweed and cook for 15 minutes. Use as a sidedish, either with sugar or vinegar and other seasoning. It can be applied for a long time.

15. Kelp

A kind of large edible alga now culti-vated artificially on a large scale.

Nature and flavour: Salt and cold.

Actions: Containing much iodine, also carrotene, vitamins B_1 and B_2 and protein.

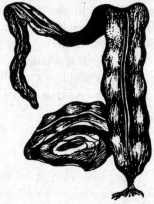

Pharmacology: The galacturonic acid in the protein has the action of lowering blood pressure. Its ether extract inhibits the growth of tuberculous bacilli.

Indicattons: Simple goiter, tuberculous lymphadenitis and chronic bronchitis in the elderly.

Recipe examples: (1) For primary hypertension. Use 60 g kelp, 150 g green bean. Boil together and add some brown sugar. Serve as tea.

(2) For tuberculous lymphadenitis. Use 7 pieces of dry lichee pulp, seaweed, and kelp, each 15 g. Put in a pot and cook in water, together with some millet wine, Chinese onion, ginger, cinnamon bark and soybean sauce, with slow fire until the kelp is well done. Serve as a side dish.

Remarks: Pregnant women are contraindicated to kelp administration.

16. Laver

A plant belonging to red alga now culti-vated artificially on a large scale.

Nature and flavour: Sweet, salty and mod-erate.

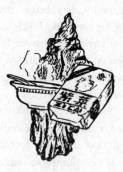

Constituents: Containing protein, fat, car-bohydrate, cellulose, carrotene, vitamins B_1, B_2 and C, iodine, calcium, phosphorus and iron. It also contains a rich amount of iodine.

Actions: Disaggregating and softening ac-tions.

Indications: For simple goitei, edema, tuberculous lymphadenitis and chronic bronchitis.

Recipe examples: For chronic bronchitis. Use 6 g dry laver to boil with 100 g *yuntun* (Chinese small dumplings stuffed with pork and shredded Chinese onion), together with some dry small shrimps (about 5 g) as soup. Then add 100 g *yuntun*. Add some soybean sauce, monosodium glutamate and a few drops of sesame oil and serve. This might be used once daily as regular meals.

B. Roots and Stems

1. Ginger

A plant belonging to the zingiberacea family. There are two kinds of ginger, the tender and the old. For medicinal use the latter is mostly applied.

Nature and flavour: Pungent and warm (the tender ginger is slightly warm).

Constituents: Ginger contains many active ingredients, including zingiberol, zingiberene, phellandrene, camphene. It has been found that gingerol is composed of shogaol and zingerone, which is the hot ingredient of ginger.

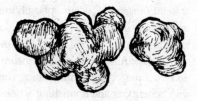

Actions: It has a biphasic action on the stomach, i.e., first inhibits its secretion and then stimulates for a longer period. It also excites the blood pressure to rise an average of 11.2 mmHg in normal people. It also yields a diaphoretic and antiemetic action. Recently it has also been found that its ingredients prevent blood coagulation, lowers blood lipides and prevents thrombosis, and is therefore very effective for preventing cardiac infarction.

Recipe examples: (1) For dysentery. Bake 30 g tender ginger and then grind into powder. Take equal amount of dry ginger powder. Mix both into flour. Add a little vinegar and prepare with minced pork as small dumplings. Serve once daily.

(2) For common cold and all kinds of vomiting. Use 10 g pounded tender ginger. Take 15 g brown sugar, dissolved in boiling water. Pour the sugar solution into the ginger and stand for a little while and drink the whole

solution. It may also be used topically. Pound 100 g old ginger and boil in water. Wash and stimulate the body skin, mainly the extremities and neck. When washing the body is needed, be sure not to catch a new cold. Avoid washing in a windy or cold room.

(3) For dyspepsia. Take 100 g tender ginger and squeeze to obtain its juice. Obtain half the amount of juice from fresh Rhizome Rehmannia. Mix them and add 2 teaspoonfuls of bee honey and boiled water. Mix thoroughly and drink as one would tea.

(4) As a stomachic and seasoning, use several slices of old or tender ginger when cooking, especially for those seafoods like fish and soft-shell turtle.

2. Lily

A plant belonging to the lily family. Both natural and domestic species serve for medicinal purposes. The bulbs are the part used.

Nature and flavour: Sweet and moderate.

Constituents: Containing protein, fat, several alkaloids and a considerable amount of starch. Calcium, phosphorus, iron, many kinds of carrotene, and several kinds of vitamins like B_1, B_2 and C are also present.

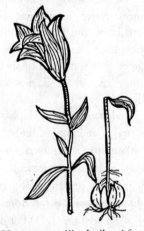

Actions: Antitussive and anti-asthmatic action. Stopping coughs, moistening the lungs with benefitting and nourishing actions.

Recipe examples: (1) For neurasthenia and nervousness. Use 7 cloves from a lily bulb and break into small pieces. Immerse in water and let stand for a whole night. Discard the water. Use 1 liter of clean water and boil to half volume. Stir thoroughly an egg's yolk and add to the water. Boil for another 5 minutes and serve. Sugar may be added.

(2) For coughing with profuse phlegm. Use 200 g lily bulb. After cleansing, toss it with some bee honey. Steam to well done and serve at any time in any amount.

3. Sweet potato

A plant belonging to the convolulacea family and widely growing throughout the country.

Nature: Sweet and moderate

Constituents: Very rich in starch and low in fat. It also contains rich carrotene, vitamins B_1, B_2 and C, calcium, and phosphorus, with a little iron.

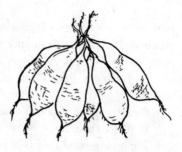

Actions: Strengthening the body, especially the spleen and stomach function. It is good for deficient kidney function and is indicated in premature ejaculation. It is also good for night blindness, best taken with animal liver, especially sheep's liver.

Remarks: Since sweet potato induces a large amount of gas in the alimentary canal, one should not eat too much at one time, or flatulence will be result. Bake sweet potato to form a brown crust or even a little bit charred. Grind it into powder. Take 3 g each time for common cold.

4. Potato

A plant belonging to the solanacea family. Its underground stem is the edible portion, the skin of which may be white, yellow or purple in colour.

Nature and flavour: Sweet and moderate.

Constituents: Containing large amounts of starch, protein, colloid material, vitamins B_1 and C, and potassium. Also containing solanin.

Actions: Its action is somewhat similar to that of sweet potato, only a little bit weaker. So, it is a splenic and stomach tonic and is good for general weakness of the body.

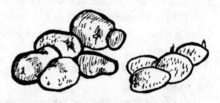

Recipe examples: (1). For general weakness and hypertension. Use 300 g potato, 100 g shallot, 4 cloves of garlic and 150 g carrot. Clean all the materials as routine but do not peel them, except for garlic. Put them in a pot and cook with slow fire until half of the water volume is gone. Add a little salt and monosodium glutamate as desired. Take one cup at the end of each meal.

(2) For peptic ulcer. Clean 1,000 g potato without peeling it first. Mince and then wrap in gauze to squeeze out juice. Then simmer this juice with very slow fire until very sticky. This potato glue is very good for relieving

pain and healing ulcers. Take a teaspoonful at each meal for a successive period of 2-3 months. Fresh juice may be also mixed with equal amount of honey for peptic ulcer. Adminster also at each meal.

(3) For burns. Potato juice may be applied topically for burns and skin eczema.

Remarks: Sprouted potato is toxic and should not be used any longer.

5. Water chestnut

The underground bulb of a plant belonging to the Cyperacea family.

Nature and flavour: Sweet and cold.

Constituents: Containing rich starch and also fat, protein, vitamin C, and puchiin.

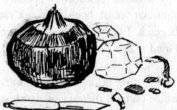

Actions: The puchiin contained in water chestnut reveals an inhibitory effect on some bacteria, especially E. coli and staphylococcus. It is good at clearing inner heat, dissolving phlegm and promoting digestive functions.

Recipe examples: (1) For clearing inner heat. Peel 100 g water chestnut. Mince to obtain its juice. Drink twice in the morning and evening. This is indicated for sore throat, stomatitis and aphtha.

(2) For bleeding in stool due to hemorrhoids. Use 500 g water chestnut. Grate it. Pour a bowl of soybean milk onto the minced water chestnut. Drink it at a draught.

(3) For jaundice. Grate 500 g water chestnut. Drink the fresh juice as one would tea.

(4) For hypertension or coughing due to heat in the lung. Clear 200 g water chestnut and 100 g jellyfish. Simmer with slow fire. Divide into 2 doses for consuming within 1 day.

6. Polygonum multiflorum (the tuber of multiflower knotweed)

Belonging to the polygonacea family. The tubers are mainly used, though its stem, termed *yejiaoteng*, is also used as a medicine.

Nature and flavour: Bitter, slightly warm.

Constituents: Containing chrysophanol, emodin, rhein, and chrysophanic acid, and anthrone. It also contains some starch and lecithin.

Actions: In animal experiments the extract of its tuber stimulates the locomotion of the intestines, and promotes the functions of digestion and absorption. It also lowers blood fats and blood sugar. So it is used as subsidiary treatment for hypertension and arteriosclerosis. In traditional Chinese medicine, it is claimed to tonify blood and vital energy, and blacken hair.

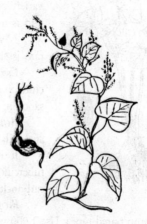

Clinical report: It was reported that 5 raw tablets, each made of 70 percent multiflower knotweed extract and 30 percent powder, was administered, thrice daily for 1/2-3 months in a group suffering hypercholenterolemia. Seventy-eight cases out of 88 showed decrease of cholesterol. However, side effect such as diarrhoea may occur, which disappeared after suspension of the tablet.

Recipe examples: (1) Use 6 g tuber of the plant and 30 g black bean. Decoct the tuber to obtain 50 ml solution. After cooking the beans separately for 1 hour, add the solutions together and cook for another 1/2 hour. Add a little salt and pork fat. Take it at a draught once daily. It is good for strengthening the body.

(2) For hypercholesterolemia. Processed tuber, 6 g infused in water and serve as one would tea, 1-2 times daily.

(3) For infirmity. Processed tuber 20 g, stoned Chinese red dates 10 pieces, 2 hen's eggs. Boil the ingredients together. After the eggs are done. Peel the shell and add some more water for further cooking. Take the water solution with the egg and dates together.

(4) For deficiency of *qi* and blood. Take 15 g processed tuber, 30-60 g rice. Prepare the rice as porridge in usual way. Decoct the tuber separately and obtain the solution which is then added to the porridge. Cook for a little while more and serve.

7. Taro

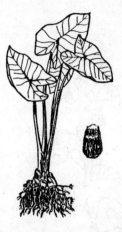

A plant belonging to the aracea family with a variety of species. Its bulb stem is edible and the raw taro is used for medical purposes.

Nature and flavour: Pungent and moderate. Raw taro is slightly toxic.

Constituents: Containing protein, fat, starch, calcium, phosphorus and iron. Also containing mucin, saponin, carrotene, and vitamins B_1, B_2 and C.

Actions: Nourishing the spleen and stomach, and anti-inflammation and analgesic actions.

It is also used in swelling of lymph nodes, tuberculous lymphadenitis. External use for boils and carbuncles, ulcers and mastitis.

Recipe examples: For tuberculous lymphadenitis (nonruptpured type). Use 1,000 g peeled taro. First cut it into small pieces in the size of strawberries and fry in vegetable oil. Then dry under sunlight and grind into powder. Use 15 g powder and dissolve in a cup of water. Sugar may be added. Administer twice a day in the morning and evening.

8. Alli macrostem's bulb

A plant belonging to the liliacea family. Its tuber root is used for medicinal and dietary purposes. Since its root is white in colour, hence the name white allium (*xiebai*) in Chinese.

Nature and flavour: Bitter, pungent and warm.

Constituents: Consisting mainly of allicin.

Actions: It is good for dispersing stagnation of *qi* and dissolving lumps and nodules, eliminating depression in stuffy chest. So, it is always used in chest distress due to coronary heart disease, angina pectoris. It is also applied in dysentery.

Recipe examples: (1) For coronary heart disease. Use 500 g bulb and clean in a usual way. Let it dry in the shadow. Immerse the whole bulb into 1 litre of vinegar contained in a bottle and add 200 g sugar.

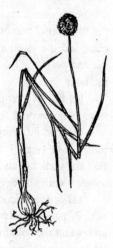

Cover the bottle tightly and let stand for half a month. By then it is ready for eating. Eat one bulb during breakfast as a side dish.

(2) Use 2 bulbs of the plant root. Wash and cut into small pieces. Prepare rice porridge in usual way. Add the shredded bulb into the porridge and boil for another 5 minutes. Serve as breakfast.

9. Chinese yam

A plant belonging to the dioscoreacea family. Its tuber root is used for medicinal purposes.

Nature and flavour: Sweet and moderate.

Constituents: Containing saponin, mucin, choline, glycoprotein, free amino acid, abscisin, etc. Also rich in starch and vitamin C.

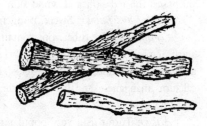

Actions: In traditional Chinese conception, yam is a very nourishing food, beneficial to the function of spleen-stomach. It is also a kidney tonic and good at preventing night emission, frequent urination due to kidney hypofunction. Also good for chronic coughing and diarrhoea. In TCM, it is always a routine remedy for diabetes mellitus.

Recipe examples: 1. For diabetes mellitus. Use 60 g yam and cut into small pieces. Take a whole piece of pig's pancreas and clean it as routine. Cook them together by slow fire until well done. Add a little salt and other flavouring materials as one likes and eat the whole thing. This might be served once daily or every other day.

2. For hypofunction of disgestion. Take 15 g yam and grate. Cook together with 50 g rice to make porridge. Use once or twice daily.

3. For anemia. Take 6 g ginseng, 30 g Chinese yam and 10 Chinese dates. With 100 g pork, cook all the materials by slow fire until the pork is well done. Serve as a draught, once a day or every other day.

4. For chronic diarrhoea. Prepare 80 g raw Chinese yam and mince. Bake another 80 g glutinous rice on a pan until a little brown. Grind the rice too and mix with the yam powder. Now add some sugar and roasted black sesame. Serve 20 g of the powder with warm boiled water every morning.

10. Turnip

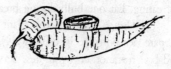

A plant belonging to the cruci-fera family, including a great variety of species, such as those with white skin, red skin, green skin with red flesh (called *xinlimei* in northern China), long shape, oval shape, etc. However, their therapeutic usage is basically the same. The tuber root and seeds are all used for medicinal purposes; the red skin and white skin species are most commonly used.

Nature and flavour: Sweet, pungent and slightly cool.

Constituents: The tuber root contains affluent water with glucose, sucrose and fructose. In addition, there are also caffeic acid, ferulic acid, benzo-pyruvic acid and many kinds of amino acids. Fresh turnip also contains vitamin C, calcium, manganese and boron. In the seeds are volatile oil, fatty acid and raphanusin.

Actions: Turnip is a very popular medicinal food. Usual consumption is very likely to bring good health. Hence, the old saying: "When turnip appears in the market the doctor is doomed to return home," and "Eat turnip in winter and ginger in summer, there's no need to trouble a doctor"; hence, the nickname "junior ginseng in the winter" for the turnip among the masses. It is usually applied in poor digestion, dispelling heat phlegm, hoarseness and bleeding. Extracts from the turnip tuber, root, as well as seeds, reveal antibacterial action. It also yields detoxified actions.

Recipe examples: (1) Abdominal flatulence or coughing with profuse phlegm. Prepare 100-200 g turnip and squeeze to obtain juice. Add 50 g rock candy and steam in water bath. Serve before bedtime for 3-5 successive nights.

(2) For chronic bronchitis. Use 200 g turnip with red skin. Cut into small pieces and put in a bowl on which 2-3 tablespoonfuls maltose are added. Let stand for a whole night. Drink the juice thus formed as one likes.

3. For uterine bleeding and other bleeding. Wash 1,000-2,000 g turnip and cut into small pieces. Squeeze to obtain 250-300 ml juice. Add 30 g sugar and divide into 2 doses. Consume in a single day.

Case example: An old man of 54 had flatulence and belching for 1 year. He felt hypofunction in his digestion and had been prescribed biofermin 2 g three times a day. He received the treatment for a period of two months to no avail.

He came to us and was advised to use the first above-mentioned recipe. His condition was markedly alleviated 2 months later and totally cured in a period of 3 months.

Remarks: Though turnip gets a nickname "minor ginseng," it is advisable not to use it together with ginseng.

11. Carrot

A plant belonging to the umbellifera family. Its seeds are also used for medicinal purposes.

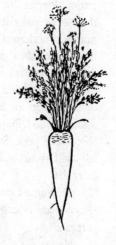

Nature and flavour: Sweet and slightly warm.

Constituents: Rich in carrotene, lycopene, sugar, fatty acid, volatile oil, vitamins B_1, B_2 and C, and umbelliferone.

Actions: Since it contains much carrotene, it is very helpful when carrots are regularly consumed, especially in preventing and treating night blindness. It is also a diuretic and stomachic, promoting digestive function.

Recipe examples: (1) For night blindness. 100 g carrot cut into slices or shreds. Stir fry under strong fire. Add salt and tender ginger filaments. Toss 100 g pig's liver into slices with corn starch powder. Stir fry in vegetable oil for a little while. Mix these two ingredients and serve as side dishes.

(2) For indigestion. Prepare 200 g carrot, 12 Chinese red dates with stones. Boil in 1,000 ml water by slow fire until 1/2 volume of water is left and serve.

(3) For impotence. Simmer carrot and dog meat in equal amount with slow fire until the meat is well done. Consume the whole thing. This recipe is better to serve in winter due to the hot nature of the meat.

(4) For anemia. Prepare 50 g carrot, 100 g spinach and 100 g lotus root. Slice carrot and lotus root. Simmer these three ingredients together for 20 minutes. Tomatoes may be used as a substitute for spinach.

12. Wild rice stem

A marine plant belonging to the graminea family. Its tender and thick rhizome is a very popular food, especially in southern China's provinces, and served as a medicine.

Nature and flavour: Sweet and cold.

Constituents: Containing protein, fat and much cellulose.

Action: This is a diuretic. It also promotes milk secretion in women after child delivery.

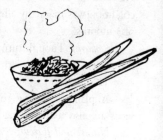

Recipe examples: (1) For promoting milk secretion. Prepare 200 g wild rice stem. Peel off its thick coats and cut into large pieces. Two pig's trotters are cleaned and treated as usual. Cook them under slow fire until the trotters are well done. Eat together in two doses.

(2) For edema. Edema is a symptom of many diseases. However, some edema is due to unknown pathogenic origins and can be treated by this medicinal food. Prepare 150 g wild rice stem as usual and slice into thin pieces. Slice 100 g pork. Stir-fry separately and then put them together. Add some salt and flavours and serve as a side dish. This might be served daily or every other day.

13. Sugar cane

A plant belonging to the graminea family. Its stem is used for medical purposes.

Nature and flavour: Sweet, moderate and slightly cold.

Constituents: In addition to affluent water, sugar, fat, and protein, there are many amino acids and minerals, such as iron and calcium. It also contains mesaconic acid, citric acid and oxalic acid, as well as vitamins B_1, B_2, B_6 and C.

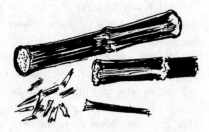

Actions: Clears heat, promotes fluid production and moistens dryness. It is very useful in febrile diseases, especially for the convalescent stage. It also stops vomiting, nausea, and coughing due to lung dryness. It is also indicated in alcoholism and constipation.

Experiments: It has been reported that the residue after squeezing out the juice contains polysaccharides, which are inhibitors to the growth of Erlich tumour and sarcoma in mice. The content is 2.6 g/2. 6 kg of residue. The cane honey produced during the process of manufacturing cane sugar also contains such polysaccharide, though in a smaller amount.

Recipe examples: (1) For febrile disease in summer. Use 500 g cane slices and boil with 50 g chrysanthemum. Serve as one would tea.

(2) For infection of urinary system manifesting frequent and urgent urination, bloody urine. Prepare 500 g fresh sugar cane, and pound to obtain its juice, 500 g lotus root. Grate and put into sugar cane juice. Then squeeze out all the juice and serve in several doses.

(3) For vomiting. A cup of juice from sugar cane, to which 8 drops of fresh ginger juice are added and serve.

Remarks: Sugar cane should be used fresh. When fungus is seen growing on its surface, it is poisonous and should not be used.

14. Lotus root

Lotus root is a plant belonging to the nymphaeacea family. All its parts are used for medicinal purposes.

Nature and flavour: Sweet, moderate and slightly cold.

Constituents: The root is rich in starch, tannate and vitamins B and C.

The stem contains alkaloid, resin and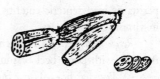
tannate. The seeds and intersegmental parts are rich in asparagin, fat, protein and starch, and the leaves are rich in nuciferine, nornuciferine, roemerine and quarcetin.

Action: Lotus seeds are nourishing and sedative. The leaves, the pod of the seeds and stem are hemostatic and astringent, while the root is a conventional hemostatic agent and helpful for thirst and fever in febrile diseases.

Recipe examples: (1) For all kinds of bleeding. Boil 500 g lotus root to obtain concentrated juice. It can be used constantly. For inner heat due to *yin* deficiency, it is also very helpful.

(2) For heat-phlegm and coughing. Prepare equal amount of juice from pear and lotus root and serve as one would tea.

(3) For dribbling urine of heat type. Prepare fresh juice from fresh lotus root, grapes and rehmanniae root. Add a little bee honey and serve as one would tea.

(4) For vomiting and thirst. Use 30 g fresh lotus root, 3 g fresh ginger. Squeeze both to obtain juice and divide it into 3 doses for daily use.

15. Onion

A very common plant belonging to the liliacea family. Its bulb stem is used for medicinal purposes.

Constituents: The constituents are rather complicated. They include thiol, methyl disulfide, allyl disulfide, allyl monosulfide and trisulfide, thiosulfinates and a little citrate, malate. Also contain caffeic acid, ferulic acid, quercetin and polysaccharide A and B and vitamins A, B_1, B_2 and C.

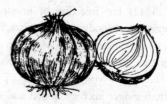

Actions: It has a bacteriocidal effect. It also lowers the cholesterol level and the activity of fibrinolysin in the blood and is therefore beneficial to coronary heart disease. It also yields some expectorant and diurectie actions.

Experiment: In model animal, it was found that onion increases the tension and secretion of intestine, so it can be applied in weak intestinal peristalsis in dysenteric enteritis. Moreover, it also excites the contraction of in vitre uterine muscles.

Recipe examples: (1) For general weakness. Consume onion constantly by frying it with pork, beef or mutton.

(2) For diarrhoea. Use 2 bulbs onion, 20 g poria. Boil them together for 15 minutes and drink at a draught.

Remarks: For people used to having flatulence, it is advisable not to use onion constantly because it may aggravate the condition.

C. Flowers, Seeds, Gourds and Fruits

1. Osmanthus flower

A flower of the osmanthus belonging to the oleacea family. It has a very strong fragrance.

Nature and flavour: Sweet, pungent and warm.

Constituents: Containing many kinds of aromatic substances, including decannolactone, ionone, linalool, nerol and geraniol.

Actions: It has an expectorant action and is able to eliminate blood stasis. So, it is always indicated in coughing asthma, toothache and bloody diarrhoea.

110

Remarks: The flowers are collected in September and October. After drying in the shadow, clean by discarding all undesired materials and parts and keep in a tightly covered container. It is commonly used when infusing tea by adding 1 g flowers into the solution. It may also be immersed in wine. Drink a little cupful each day for all pains of cold type.

2. Chrysanthemum

There are many varieties of chrysanthemum, of which only some species are used for medicinal purposes. It is mainly made into a tea-like drink.

Nature and flavour: Bitter, sweet and moderate.

Actions: In traditional Chinese medicine, it is claimed that chrysanthemum clears fever and eliminates evil dampness, relieves dizziness and improves eyesight.

Constituents: Contains volatile oil and adenine, choline and stachydrine. It also contains chrysanthemun aminoacids and borneol.

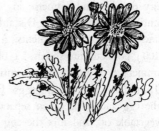

Actions: It was found that chrysanthemum yields bacteriocidal effect and antiviral effect in high concentration. So, it is always indicated in primordial stage of fever. It reveals an action of strengthening the resistance of capillaries and some anti-inflammatory actions. It also relieves dizziness, improves eyesight to some extent, and is always applied for hypertension.

Recipe examples: (1) For dizziness. Use 10 g dry chrysanthemum flower and immerse in wine. Drink daily as one likes.

(2) For hypertension. Take chrysanthemum and green tea, each 3 g to

make tea infusion with boiling water as one would tea. This may be applied on a daily basis for a long period.

(3) For primordial stage of cold or flu. Use chrysanthemum and mulberry leaves (dry or fresh) in equal amount, infuse with boiling water and use as tea.

3. Day lily

In China, it is also called yellow-flower vegetable and belongs to the liliacea family.

Nature and flavour: Sweet and cool.

Constituents: Containing asparagin, colchicine, vitamins A, B and C, protein and anthra-quinone A, B, C, D and F.

Action: Anti-inflammation, antipyretic and analgesic. Also having diuretic action and relieving deep-coloured urine in children.

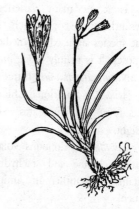

Recipe examples: (1) For all kinds of mild bleeding. Use 10 g root of day lily decocted in 100 ml water under slow fire for 15 minutes and serve as one would tea.

(2) For general infirmity. Prepare 20 g dry day lily and immerse in warm water until it becomes tender. Discard hard ends and cut into small segments. Also prepare 100 g pork cut into shreds, 5 g black fungus immersed in warm water until softened. Thoroughly stir 2 hen's eggs. First stir-fry the egg and pork. Then separately fry the other ingredients together with vegetable oil, and mix the egg and add some other flavourings. Serve as a side dish. It can be applied constantly.

(3) Pound 50 g fresh day lily and apply topically for boils, carbuncles or mastitis.

4. Tomato

A plant belonging to the solanacea family with special odour.

Nature and flavour: Sour, slightly sweet and moderate.

Constituents: Containing large amounts of water, vitamins C, B_1 and B_2, calcium, phosphorus, iron, adenine, choline, trigenelline, carrotene and a small quantity of tomatine.

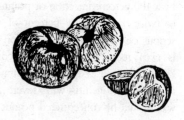

Actions: Tomatine is effective in inhibiting fungus infection in human body. It also possesses some anti-inflammatory action and decreases the permeability of blood vessels. Animal experiments also reveal that it temporarily lowers blood pressure, but with no effect on heart rate. In traditional Chinese medicine, it is claimed that tomato possesses antipyretic and detoxicated actions.

Recipe examples: (1) For common cold in summer with loss of appetite, restlessness, thirst and deep-coloured urine. Use equal amount of tomato and watermelon and obtain its juice. Mix the two kinds of juice together and drink as one likes.

(2) For hypertension. Consume 2 fresh tomatoes in the morning with empty stomach each day for a period of 1-2 months.

(3) For night blindness. Prepare 250 g fresh tomato, 60 g pig's liver. Slice the liver and toss with a little corn starch or sweet potato starch. First fry the liver in vegetable oil and add some soybean sauce. Add the sliced tomato together with a little monosodium glutamate and serve as a side dish.

5. Peanut

A plant belonging to the leguminosa family.

Nature and flavour: Sweet and moderate.

Constituents: Containing large amounts of fat, also vitamins A, B, E and K, lecithin, choline, betaine, purine, arachine, amino acids, calcium, etc.

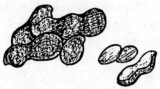

Actions: Experiments demonstrate that peanuts with its membranous skin shortens the coagulation time of human blood and so it is apt for hemophilia. Its oil lowers blood pressure and the contents of blood cholesterol. It was found that the membranbus skin is even more effective than the peanut itself.

Clinical reports: A total of 285 cases of various hemorrhages were treated by a 100 percent injection of peanut skin injected intramuscularly 2-5 ml once or twice daily. Eighty percent of the cases revealed satisfactory effects. For serious cases, intravenous injection can be applied. It was emphasized that it is even more effective for bleeding due to cancers, surgical operations, hemophilia and idiopathic purpura hemorrhagica. Another group of 407 cases of chronic bronchitis with severe asthmatic coughing with profuse sputum was treated by concentrated peanut skin solution for a course of 10 days. Of them 230 cases were ameliorated, 74 markedly effective and 8 cases brought under control, an effective rate of 76.6 percent.

Recipe examples: (1) For hemophilia and purpura. Prepare 250 g peanuts with skin intact, 15 g Chinese dates with stones discarded, 12 g dry longan pulp. Boil all ingredients in water with slow fire until peanuts are well done. Consume all the residue and decoction, once daily.

(2) For dry coughing, pertusis (whooping cough). Boil 50 g rock sugar in water until the syrup becomes sticky and can be rendered into filaments. Add 250 g fried peanuts and mix thoroughly. Pour into a container with its wall rubbed with oil in advance. Press the mass to form small pieces of candy and eat as one likes.

(3) For promoting lactation after child birth. Thoroughly clean a pig's front trotter. Add 30 g peanuts and simmer with slow fire until both are well done. Eat both ingredients and drink its soup.

Remarks: Peanuts are susceptible to contamination of aflatoxin produced by a fungus, aspergillus flavus, which is very toxic and carcinogenic, especially a risk factor to liver carcinoma. Once the peanut reveals a greenish yellow appearance, it is dangerous and can no longer be used.

6. Red bean

A plant belonging to the leguminosa family. The whole bean is red in colour and easy to distinguish from the jequirity bean which, though similar in shape, is half red and half black and is toxic.

Nature and flavour: Sweet and moderate.

Constituents: Containing starch, protein and fat, ormosanine, piptanthine, vitamins A, B and C, saponin, aluminium and copper.

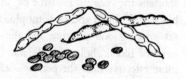

Actions: It possesses diuretic action and is indicated in edema and diarrhoea. It is an antidote in Chinese medicine and used to be applied in boils, carbuncles, erysipelas, and bloody stool which are believed to be the results of poisons.

Recipe examples: (1) For mumps. Pound 50 g red beans and prepare as powder. Add some honey and a little warm water to make paste for local application.

(2) For abdominal pain after child delivery. Fry 300 g red beans until a little bit charred. Boil in 500 ml by slow fire until half of its volume is gone. Add some brown sugar. Drink in 3 equal doses in a day.

7. Hyacinth bean

A plant belonging to the leguminosa family.

Nature and flavour: Sweet and slightly warm.

Constituents: Containing protein, fat and sugar. Also with pantothenic acid, calcium, phosphorus, iron, zinc and phytin.

Actions: It strengthens the spleen-stomach, eliminates dampness and summer heat and is mostly applied in hypofunction of spleen-stomach, edema, diarrhoea and scanty, deep-coloured urine. It also is indicated for leucorrhea due to evil dampness.

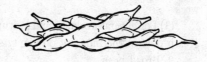

Recipe examples: (1) For leucor-rhea due to evil dampness as a result of deficient spleen. Use 50 g hyacinth bean. Immerse it in water from washing rice until the beans are swollen. Peel the beans. Put in water and boil with 30 g brown sugar, 15 g poria until the beans are well cooked. Consume the beans, poria and the soup.

. (2) For sunstroke. Use 15 g hyacinth bean, 6 g Herba Elsholtziae seu Moslae, with half sheet of lotus leaf. Boil together until the beans are well done. Filter with the residue discarded and drink the filtrate. Add some sugar as one likes.

(3) For edema. Use 200 g hyacinth bean. Immerse in rice-washing water and remove the peels. After drying in the shadow, fry it. Make powder with this bean. Eat 3 g, twice a day in the morning and evening.

Remarks: In dealing with hyacinth bean, be sure to cook it thoroughly and well done. Beans not well done are poisonous.

8. Cowpea

A plant belonging to the leguminosa family.

Nature and flavour: Sweet, salty and moderate.

Constituents: Containing starch, fat and protein. Also containing nicotinic acid, vitamins B_1, B_2 and C.

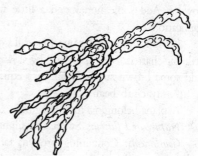

Actions: It strengthens the spleen and nourishes the kidney and is applied in diarrhoea due to deficient spleen and dyspepsia. It is also applied in leucorrhoea, frequent urine and night emission.

Recipe examples: (1) For dyspepsia with flatulence. Raw cowpea is chewed or pounded and swallowed with cooled boiled water.

(2) For leucorrhoea. Prepare cowpea and water spinach, each 100 g, and simmer with a chicken until well done. This can be served once or twice a week.

(3) For general weakness and polyuria. Boil cowpea for daily use, 150-300 g each dose in the morning on empty stomach.

9. Broad bean

A plant belonging to the leguminosa family.

Nature and flavour: Sweet, slightly pungent and moderate.

Constituents: Containing protein, fat and carbohydrate, vicine, choline, lecithin, pipecolic acid, amino acid, vitamins B_1 and B_2.

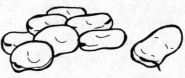

Actions: It strengthens spleen and expels evil dampness as well as hemostatic action, and is applied in hemorrhage, edema, and diarrhoea due to deficient spleen. It also inhibits some fungus infection of the head (favus of the scalp).

Recipe examples: (1) For edema. Prepare 200-400 g broad beans, and 500 g beef. Simmer with slow fire until well done and serve. This can be applied once or twice a week. But the recipe should not include spinach.

(2) For tinea capitis (scalp favus). Pound sufficient amount of broad beans and apply the crushed beans topically to the affected region on the scalp. Fresh beans are preferable, but dried beans can be used if former unavailable.

(3) For difficult swallowing. Use 500 g dried broad beans and grind as powder. Mix with brown sugar. Administer once in the morning on empty stomach.

(4) For stopping bleeding and diarrhoea. Prepare broad bean powder with dry specimen. Dissolve 10 g in water, 3 times a day.

Remarks: Vicine contained in broad bean may cause allergic reactions in some people, especially young males. The manifestations are bloody urine, dizziness, vomiting or even jaundice. This condition is called favism, occurring on the basis of congenital defect and should be treated in time.

10. Black bean

A plant belonging to the leguminosa family. Its wild species called *Maliao* bean is best for medicinal uses.

Nature and flavour: Sweet and moderate.

Constituents: Containing fat, protein and sugar, vitamins B_1, B_2 and B_{12}, carrotene, nicotinic acid, daidzin, daidzein, soyasapogenol, choline, biotin and minerals, such as potassium, iron. The protein contained in black bean is higher (49.8 percent) than regular soyabean.

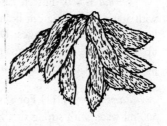

Actions: It passesses some diuretic and detoxicated actions. In traditional Chinese conception, it blackens the hair by its kidney nourishing potential. By the same action, it also expels edema and evil dampness.

Recipe examples: (1) For blackening hair. Boil 500 g black beans in 1 litre vinegar until well done. Discard the residue and continue to boil by slow fire to obtain a concentrated solution. Use 10 ml as shampoo for washing hair. Meanwhile, take 20 pieces of fried black bean each evening with a teaspoonful of fried black sesame.

(2) For postpartum pain over the body. Fry 250 g black beans to brown and immerse in millet wine for a whole day. Drink 10 ml wine and sleep

with quilt to obtain slight sweat.

(3) For nourishing the kidney *yin*. Prepare 500 g dog meat and 50 g black beans. Clean both as usual and then simmer with slow fire until all are well done. Divide this into 12 equal portions and eat 1-2 portions daily. This is good for senile deafness and sterility due to deficient kidney.

11. Green bean

A plant belonging to the leguminosa family.

Nature and flavour: Sweet and cold.

Constituents: Containing globulins, fat, starch, vitamins carrotene B_1 and B_2, calcium, phosphorus iron, and phosphaticly-lethanolamine and other phosphorus compounds.

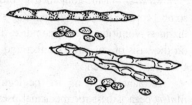

Actions: In ancient China, green bean was extensively applied as an antidotes for all kinds of poisoning. It also clears heat with dampness expelling actions. So, it is used for anti-summer heat, edema, diarrhoea and boils and carbuncles.

Clinical reports: Fifteen cases of pesticide 1,059 poisoning were treated with 500 g pounded green beans and 10 g salt immersed in 2 litres of cooled boiled water for 15 minutes. Drink as much of the filtrate as possible, even up to 3 litres. In comatous patient, infusion through nasal feeding was performed. All the cases were cured within 24 hours. Green bean curd may also be used.

Recipe examples: (1) For summer heat stroke. Boil 100 g green beans in 500 ml water with strong fire, and drink after cooling down. The residue can also be consumed.

(2) For dysuria. Take 500 g green bean and 60 g tangerine peel. Boil together in water until the beans are well done. Add some drops of sesame oil and drink on empty stomach.

(3) For bloody stool. Use 50 g crushed cannabis sativa. Immerse in water and filter. Boil another 50 g green beans in the filtrate. Rice may be added to make porridge.

12. Soybean

A plant belonging to the leguminosa family.

Nature and flavour: Sweet, moderate and slightly cold.

Constituents: Basically the same as that of black bean, only the protein content is a little less (40 percent) than the latter. Since it is far more popularly consumed in daily life, it 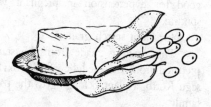 wins the title, "vegetarian meat." Soybean sauce and a great variety of bean curd products in traditional Chinese daily use is made of this bean.

Actions: It is mostly applied to strengthen the body, such as for anemia, infirmity, antipoisoning, promoting lactation, leucorrhoea and asthma. Its derivatives, including soybean milk, bean curd and bean sprout are ideal remedies for general weakness.

Clinical application: Ninety-two cases of eclampsia were treated with pure soybean curd (1:8 in water). 100 g sugar and 1 bowl (200 ml) of curd were given 6 times a day. The patients were banned from salt. From the 2nd day, fruits may be given. Forty-one cases were treated with routine Western therapies. No mortality was seen in the bean curd group, while that for the control group was 2.43 percent. The satisfactory result was attributed to high vitamin B_1, nicotinic acid and water, low calcium, sodium, resulting in lowering of blood pressure and diuresis.

Recipe examples: (1) For common cold. Prepare a handful of soybean, 3 segments of Chinese onion bulb, one cabbage "head," 5 slices of white turnip. Decoct all the ingredients for 15 minutes and drink the decoction at a draught. It is good for both treatment and prevention.

(2) For bronchial asthma. Take 500 g bean curd and a cup of fresh turnip juice. Boil and consume all of them in a draught. It may be administered for several days.

(3) For leucorrhoea. Crush 10 gingko and put it into 200 ml bean milk. Boil and drink up. It can be served for several days.

(4) For habitual constipation. Use 200 g membranous skin of soybean. Decoct in 200 ml water and drink in 3 equal parts in a single day.

(5) For diarrhoea. Bake the membranous skin of soybean charred and use 3-9 g each time. Swallow with boiled water twice a day.

Remarks: Soybean sprout is sweet, moderate and cold. Sprout soup is good for hypertension in pregnant women, and coughing with yellow sputum.

13. Palm starch grain

This grain is made from the starch prepared from the medulle of Metroxylon sagu Rottb, a plant belonging to the palm family.

Nature and flavour: Sweet, moderate and warm.

Constituents: Mainly composed of starch.

Actions: Strengthening the spleen, warming the interior, benefitting the lungs and eliminating sputum.

Indications: Deficiency of the spleen-stomach functions, dyspepsia of deficient-cold type. Weakness due to severe illness or postpartum.

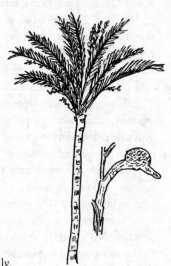

14. Husked sorghum

A grain belonging to the graminea family.

Nature and flavour: Sweet and slightly cold.

Constituents: Mainly composed of fat, protein, starch and protosugar.

Action: Effective for insomnia coupled with dyspesia due to weakness of the spleen-stomach functions.

Recipe examples: (1) For dyspepsia in children. Use 50 g red sorghum and 10 Chinese red dates. Discard the date stones and bake all together to brown. Grind as powder.

Dosage: 10 g, twice daily. It was reported that 104 cases were treated with the recipe. A hundred cases were cured within only 2 days; only the remaining 4 failed.

(2) For diarrhoea. Use the sorghum pow-

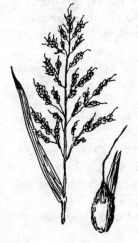

der prepared as in the above recipe. Swallow with boiled water.

15. Maize

A plant belonging to the graminea family.

Nature and flavour: Sweet and moderate.

Constituents: Mainly fatty acid, volatile oil, resin, zeaxanthin, carrotene, zeatin, saponin, alkaloids. The seeds contain protein, vitamins B_1, B_2, B_6 and E, calcium, phosphorus and iron.

Actions: It may lower blood pressure and blood sugar. It is also a hemostatic. Its diuretic action is extrarenal in nature.

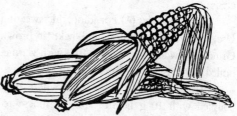

Recipe examples: (1) For edema in nephritis. Prepare long hairs from maize, external skin of white (wax) gourd and red bean, each 20 g. Infuse in boiling water for several minutes and drink as one would tea.

(2) For night sweats. Use 60 g hard kernel of maize and 30 g oyster shell. Pound as powder and boil for 15 minutes. Drink the decoction, once daily.

(3) For diuresis. Boil 30 g fresh maize leaves with slow fire for 20 minutes. Drink the soup once daily.

Remarks: Oil from maize is a good remedy for lowering blood cholesterol.

16. Wheat

A plant belonging to the graminea family, the staple food in North China. Floating wheat refers to those dry and shrivelled grains which float on the surface of water.

Nature and flavour: Sweet and slightly cold.

Constituents: Containing protein, starch, saccharin, fat, cellulose, ergosteriod, lecithin, allantoin, amylase and vitamin B.

Actions: Beneficial to the heart and mind, relieving perspiration due to asthenia. Also good for boils and carbuncles.

Clinical report: It was reported that old wheat is good for skin infections.

Use 1,000 g old wheat (produced at least in the previous year or even older). Add 3,000 ml water and immerse the wheat for 3 days. Pound the immersed wheat. Filter. Let the filtrate stand and then use its precipitate. Add vinegar to the precipitate to form a paste for external application. Effective for erysipelas, boils and carbuncles.

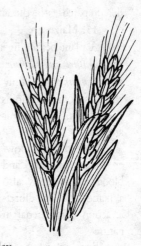

Recipe examples: (1) For idiopathic sweating. Use some floating wheat and bake it brown. Grind as powder and swallow 10 g with warmed boiled water twice or thrice a day.

(2) For hysteria. Boil 30 g wheat grain coupled with 10 g licorice and 5 Chinese red dates in water. Consume the whole thing, once a day.

(3) For insomnia. Boil 60 g wheat grain, 25 pieces of Chinese red dates, 15 g licorice in 500-600 ml water with slow fire until 250 ml is left. Drink in 2 equal doses in the morning and evening.

17. Barley

A plant belonging to the graminea family. Its sprout is used for medicinal purposes.

Nature and flavour: Salty and warm.

Constituents: Containing maltose, glucose, saccharin, lecithin, allantoin, amylase and vitamin B.

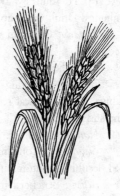

Actions: Benefiting the functions of spleen and stomach, and relieving dyspepsia. Eliminating dampness to promote urination.

Recipe examples: (1) For summer heat. The use of barley as a substitute for tea in summer is good for preventing summer heat stroke. Fry 50 g barley to slightly brown. Infuse in boiling water and add a few slices of ginger.

(2) For diuresis. Prepare 100 g barley and boil with 200 ml water for 10 minutes. Then

drop several drops of fresh ginger juice and drink before meals.

18. Rice

The kernel of the seeds of the plant rice, belonging to the grominea family. It may be husked or unhusked.

Nature and flavour: Sweet and moderate (warm when produced in northern China).

Constituents: Rich in starch (over 75 percent) with a little protein and some vitamin B, glucose, surcrose and maltose.

Actions: In traditional Chinese concept, it has long been claimed that rice strengthens the spleen-stomach and stops diarrhoea. The porridge made of rice is believed to be the most powerful tonic of all. It is especially suitable for the aged, infirm, postpartal women, and patients at the convalescent stage. Sprouted rice is very helpful to digestion. Experiments also demonstrated that old glutinous rice stored for over 3 years with contaminated and grown microbes can be baked at 80°C and then prepared as water suspension with extracts in water or in ethyl alcohol. This recipe possesses potential to inhibit tumour growth in animals.

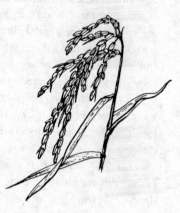

Recipe examples: (1) For chronic diarrhoea with loss of appetite. Immerse 250 g rice in cold water for a whole night. Then discard the water and bake to well done under slow fire and grind as powder. Add 5 g poria powder and mix thoroughly. Administer 30-40 g with sugar and pepper in small amounts.

(2) For infirmity. Prepare 60 g powdered rice to which cinnamon bark, prickly ash, Fructus Amomi, each 6 g, are added. All ingredients are mixed and pounded as powder. Drink 6 g with warmed boiled water, 3 times daily.

(3) For dyspepsia. Use 500 g rice crust (the brown hard portion around the wall and at the bottom of the pot), 100 g scorched hawthorn, 200 g Chinese yam, and 50 g Fructus Amomi. All ingredients are prepared as powder. Dosage is 10 g taken with some sugar, twice each day.

(4) For diarrhoea due to hypofunction of the spleen. Prepare 100 g

glutinous rice, 30 g lotus seeds, 20 pieces Chinese red dates and 15 g poria. Clean all ingredients as usual and boil together with slow fire until rice is well done. Add suitable amount of sugar, and serve as regular meals.

19. Chestnut

A plant belonging to the fagacea family. It may be domestic or wild. Its fruit is used for medicinal purposes.

Nature and flavour: Sweet and warm.

Constituents: Rich in starch and sugar, protein, fat, and vitamins B_1 and B_2, fat and enzymes (lipase).

Actions: Chestnut reveals tonic action on many aspects, including spleen, stomach and kidneys. It also regulates the disharmonized and adverse flowing of *qi* in the body. Also applied in bleeding.

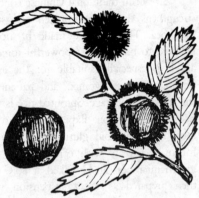

Recipe examples: (1) For itching pharynx and throat. Use 5-10 pieces of shelled raw chestnut for chewing.

(2) For weakness in lower limbs. Prepare 100 g chestnut (fresh or dry) and boil in water. Add appropriate amount of brown sugar. Eat several pieces before bedtime.

(3) For polyuria or frequent urination due to hypofunction of kidneys. The same recipe can be given as for weak limbs stated above.

(4) Infantile diarrhoea. Prepare 50 g persimmon cake (dried persimmon) and 30 g shelled crushed chestnut. Mix thoroughly to form a jelly-like mixture. Steam and serve.

20. Fruit of Chinese wolfberry

A plant belonging to the solanacea family. Its tender leaves are edible and the fruit is used as a medicinal food.

Nature and flavour: Sweet and moderate.

Constituents: Containing nicotinic acid, carrotene, vitamins B_1, B_2 and C, zeaxanthin, betaine, physalien, ß-ergosteriod and lenoleic acid.

Actions: It possesses an action antagonistic to fat deposition, especially in the liver. So it is often applied in obese patients and in liver disease with lipidosis. It lowers the level of blood sugar and is beneficial to diabetes. It also nourishes the *yin* principle and blood, and improves one's eyesight.

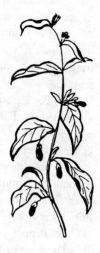

Experimental results: It was demonstrated that this fruit yields a prominent action in protecting the liver from lipid accumulation. When mice were poisoned with CCl_4 in the laboratory, those receiving administration of extracts from this fruit yielded no liver function impairment, while the control group, which received no protection, were mostly poisoned and killed.

Recipe examples: (1) For general weakness due to deficient kidney, manifesting impaired eyesight, dizziness, impotence, weak waist and knee. Immerse 30-60 g fruit of Chinese wolfberry in 60 percent liquor for at least 7 days (the longer, the better). Drink 5-10 ml each day.

(2) For the aged and infirm. Prepare 25 g fruit to make rice porridge. Use porridge as a regular meal once or twice daily.

(3) For diabetes mellitus. Prepare 15 g fruit, 250 g rabbit meat and cook it under slow fire until the meat is well done. Add salt and flavouring and serve as a side dish.

21. Fructus Amomi

An aromatic flavouring produced from a plant belonging to the zingiberacea family.

Nature and flavour: Pungent and warm.

Constituents: Volatile oil, d-camphor, bornyl acetate, d-Borneol, nerolidol, linalool, etc.

Actions: It is warm and promotes *qi* flowing in its right track. It is applied in epigastric distention, flatulence, belching, nausea, vomiting and loss of appetite.

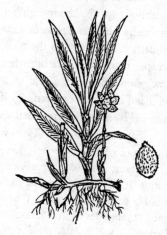

Recipe examples: (1) For stomach ache

due to deficient spleen and stomach as well as gastroptosis. Prepare a pig's stomach and rinse it thoroughly. Fill the interiors with 6 g Fructus Amomi, 20 g root of membranous milk vetch. Cook it first with strong fire and then with slow fire until it is thoroughly well done. Discard the residue of the fruits and roots. Add salt and flavourings and consume the stomach and the soup.

(2) For infantile anal prolapse. Use a few powdered Fructus Amomi and a pig's kidney. Eliminate all the white tissues and then toss it with the wet powder. Cut into several pieces and cook. Add flavouring to the cooked kidney and serve.

(3) For distention in the chest due to internal phlegm. Drink of Fructus Amomi and turnip: Crush 6 g Fructus Amomi. Cut 500 g turnip into thin slices. Boil both together and divide the decoction into 3 equal parts. Administer it hot half an hour after each meal.

22. Pepper

There are two kinds of pepper, black and white, both belonging to the piperacea family and yielding similar actions.

Nature and flavour: Pungent and hot.

Constituents: Containing piperine, chavicine, piperonal, piperanine, cryptone, caryophyllene oxide, etc.

Actions: Due to its hot nature, pepper is good for expelling evil cold and warming up the body interior, especially when cold phlegm accumulates and stagnates in the body. Pepper is also a stomachic when one's stomach suffers a cold invasion and is in need of warming. It also yields some antipyretic action.

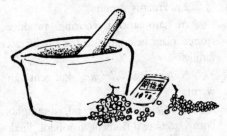

Experimental results: Twenty-four cases of healthy people were researched by keeping 0.1 g pepper under the tongue. The blood pressure was examined before and after the experiments. It was discovered that there was temporary rise of blood pressure (18.1 mmHg for systolic and 13.1 mmHg for diastolic pressure) with recovery to pre-examined levels 10-15 minutes later. There was no change in pulse rate. Pepper also stimulates the involuntary movements of isolated intestinal and uterine muscles of animals in vitro.

Recipe examples: (1) For vomiting due to cold in the stomach. Immerse some pepper in vinegar. Then take it out and dry under sunlight. Repeat the process 7 times. Grind the pepper into powder. Administer 3 g, twice daily.

(2) For cold of wind-cold type. Prepare pepper and clove, each 3 g. Grind them as powder. Use 2 white bulbs from Chinese onion and pound, then mix with the prepared powder. Put a small mass onto the palm. Close both palms together and put the closed hands in between the two thighs until one sweats.

(3) For dyspepsia in children. Grind 1 g white pepper as powder and 9 g glucose powder. Mix them together. Administer 0.3-0.8 g (< 1 year old), 0.5-1.5 g (< 3 years old), thrice daily, 1-3 days for a therapeutic course.

(4) For prolapse of stomach. Clean a pig's or sheep's stomach (about 500 g) to which 1.5 g white pepper is added. Simmer with slow fire until well done. Consume the stomach and soup.

Remarks: For people used to have flaring up of inner fire, manifesting red eyes, sore throat or thirst, pepper is contraindicated.

23. Chilli

A plant belonging to the solanacea family, with a great variety of species different in shape and with different quantities of chilli elements.

Nature and flavour: Pungent and warm.

Constituents: Capsaicin, capsanthin, fatty oil, solasodine, solanidine, solanine and considerable amount of vitamin C.

Actions: The chillic ingredients contained in chilli stimulates appetite and is a stomachic when used in an appropriate amount. It is a very useful flavour. The species containing no chillic ingredients is a very rich source of vitamin C. It also yields some antibacterial effect.

Experimental results: When appropriate quantity of chilli is administered, it stimulates the membrane of digestive tract to secrete digestive juices and promote digestion. When the hot ingredient stimulates the taste buds in the tongue, through reflex action, blood pressure (mainly diastolic), rises, but no changes in pulse rate

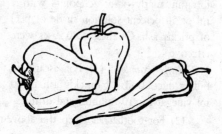

were observed.

Clinical reports: When a paste containing chilli powder, vaseline and millet wine, was applied topically to tender points on the waist and lower extremities, the pain in 1 case was cured, 25 cases alleviated, 23 markedly effective, the effective rate being 75.4 percent. For frostbite, 200 cases were treated topically by washing with chilli solution boiled for 3-5 minutes with 50-100 g tender wheat seedlings, once daily. All the cases but 4 were cured.

Recipe examples: (1) For common cold. Boil 3 pieces of chilli, 10 pieces of Chinese prickly ash, 1 slice of ginger and a little salt. Drink the decoction and keep warm.

(2) For cold abdominal pain and water diarrhoea. 1 g powdered chilli wrapped with a sheet of skin from soybean curd. Swallow with warmed boiled water.

(3) For baldness. Immerse 10 g minced dry chilli in liquor for 7 days. Wash the affected scalp with this lotion.

24. Chinese prickly ash

A plant belonging to the rutacea family.

Nature and flavour: Pungent and warm.

Constituents: Volatile oil, mainly composed of limonene, cumic alcohol and geraniol; steriod and unsaturated organic acid.

Actions: The active ingredients from prickly ash yield some analgesic or anesthetic action. For instance, diluted alcoholic solution of prickly ash reveals local surface anesthesis of cornea in rabbit. It also showed infiltrative analgesic action in guinea pig.

Clinical reports: 246 cases of acute abdomen, including peptic ulcer, intestinal spasm, biliary cholic were injected intramuscularly or at acupoints with 2 ml of 50 percent solution made of peel of prickly ash. Of these, 240 cases were effective.

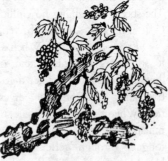

Recipe examples: (1) For ascaris in biliary duct. Boil 3 g prickly ash in 60 ml vinegar for 10 minutes and drink.

(2) For toothache. Keep the above-mentioned decoction in mouth for

several minutes.

(3) For cold stomach ache and nausea. Boil 2 g prickly ash and 6 g old ginger in water. Add some brown sugar and then administer.

25. Aniseed

A plant belonging to the magnoliacea family.

Nature and flavour: Pungent, warm and sweet.

Constituents: It contains 3-6 percent volatile oil, mainly composed of anethole, fenchone, α-pinene, anise aldehyde, anisic acid and estragole.

Actions: It invigorates the movements of alimentary tract, expelling the excess gas out of the canal. Hence, it is mainly used for relieving intestinal spasm and stopping its pain. It also stops pain of other kinds like hernia, menstrual, and scrotal pains.

Clinical reports: Twenty-six cases of strangulated hernia in children with a course from 2 hours to 3 days were treated with hot aniseed decoction (9-15 g decocted in water). The patients adopted a supine position with lower limbs close together and knees slightly bent. Twenty-two cases were thus cured.

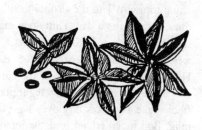

Recipe examples: (1) For intestinal hernia. Bake 40 g aniseed and then grind as powder. Dissolve 5 g in warm boiled water and drink at a draught.

(2) For lumbago. Fry 50 g aniseed and then grind into powder. Use 6 g powdered aniseed with a little salt in warmed boiled water on empty stomach, twice daily.

(3) For scrofulia. Prepare 15 g aniseed with 4.5 g salt by first frying together and then grind as powder. Stir 2 hen's eggs and mix the powder with the eggs to make pies. Eat the pie with some millet wine before bedtime, once daily for 4 days.

(4) For stomach ache of cold type. Boil 10 g aniseed in water for 10 minutes and then add some brown sugar. Drink the decoction.

Remarks: Patients with red eyes or skin troubles should avoid aniseed.

26. Clove

A tropical plant belonging to the myrtacea family.

Nature and flavour: Pungent and warm.

Constituents: Clove oil in the buds contains mainly eugenol, eugenin euginone, humulene and chavicol.

Action: It possesses some inhibitory effect on bacteria. Stomachic and stops toothache. In traditional Chinese medicine, it is claimed that it warms the spleen and stomach and stops vomiting, and hiccups due to evil coldness of stomach.

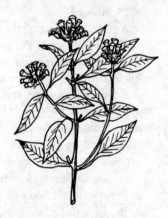

Clinical reports: Clove was used for tinea of the skin and revealed satisfactory effects, by immersing 15 g in 100 ml of 70 percent alcohol for 48 hours and administering topically. Use the alcohol to rub skin tinea, three times a day. Thirty-one cases of skin tinea with a history of over 2 years were thus treated. Generally, 3-5 days of treatment is enough to cure. However, about 20 percent of the cured cases relapsed repeatedly.

Recipe examples: (1) For regurgitation of milk in infants with greenish stool. Take 10 pieces of clove, 3 g old tangerine peel with 1 cup of human milk. Boil together and feed the infant slowly, bit by bit.

(2) For vomiting and diarrhoea in infants. Decoct 2 g clove, 3 g dry tangerine peel for 10 minutes. Then add some bee honey and feed the patient.

(3) For stomach ache of cold type. Decoct 1.5 g clove and 1 g cinnamon bark in water. Add brown sugar to the decoction, three times a day.

27. Olive

The fruit of a plant belonging to the burseracea family.

Nature and flavour: Sweet, sour and warm.

Constituents: It contains protein, fat, sugar, vitamin C, calcium, phosphorus, iron, volatile oil and amyrin.

Actions: Nourishing body fluids and detoxification, eliminating sputum and good for sore throat.

Clinical reports: It was reported that olive was effective for acute bacillary dysentery and tinea dermatosis. For dysentery, put 100 g olive with the kernel in an earthenware pot and add 200 ml water. Cook with slow fire for 2-3 hours until half volume of water is evaporated. Use the solution 3-4 times daily until normal stool appears. Forty-nine cases were cured clinically with fever subsiding 12 hours after administration. For eczema, acute dematitis with exudates, pound the stoned olive and apply it locally. These results were also satisfactory.

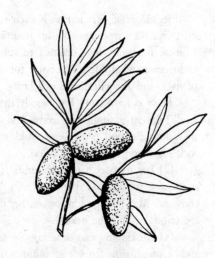

Recipe examples: (1) For sore throat. Keep a fresh or preserved olive in the mouth and swallow the saliva bit by bit. For preserving the olive, just add salt to the olives after drying in the shadow for 1-2 days. Use an earthenware vessel. After a period of 2 weeks, preserved olives are ready for use. The stones inside the olive may be removed or preserved intact.

(2) For alcoholism. Pound 5-10 fresh olives. Use 200 ml water, add 40 g sugar and boil for 15 minutes. Consume the solution. Repeat when necessary.

(3) For chronic coughing. Use 5 pitted fresh olives and mix with rock sugar in appropriate amount. Steam for half an hour.

28. Sunflower

A plant belonging to the composita family. Its seed dish, flower and stem are all used for medicinal purposes.

Nature and flavour: Sweet, warm and moderate.

Constituents: The oil from its seeds contains glyceride and linolenic acid, ß-sitosterol. Its stem contains polysaccharide and chlorogenic acid.

Actions: Animal experiments reveal that the oil from sunflower seeds prevents hyperlipidemia and hypercholesterolemia, though experiments in man with its crude oil may result in a temporary rise of blood cholesterol. When the flower disk is prepared as paste by boiling in water, it is effective for arthritis when applied locally. It also exerts certain effects on hypertension when the disk is prepared as syrup.

131

Its alcoholic preparation is even more effective for hypertension. In traditional Chinese medicine, it is claimed to subdue endogenous wind due to excessive function of liver, and also eliminates evil heat.

Recipe examples: (1) For bloody dysentery. Take 50 g sunflower seeds. Add 500 ml water and boil for 1 hour. Add some rock sugar and drink the solution.

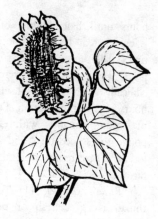

(2) For measles. Crush the nuts from sunflower seeds. Add boiling water and consume. May be repeated for another dose the same day and the next day.

(3) For ringing ears. Pound 30 g sunflower seeds. Add some rock sugar and boil with slow fire for 30 minutes. Drink the whole solution twice a day.

29. Seeds of Job's-tears

The seeds are from a plant belonging to the graminea family.

Nature and flavour: Sweet and slightly cold.

Constituents: Sugar, fat, protein, coixol, coixenolide and triterpenes.

Actions: Benefitting the spleen functions, eliminating edema, diuretic and nourishing the digestive functions.

Experimental results: In experiments in rats, coixol revealed actions antagonistic to caffeine, i.e. inhibition to the central nervous system, with some antipyretic and analgesic effect. It has also been reported that the seeds yield some anticancer effect.

Clinical reports: It was reported that Job's-tears also inhibit the growth of warts. A group of 23 cases were treated by Job's-tears porridge by boiling 50 g Job's-tears plus 50 g rice together. This was administered once daily. After 7-16 days, 11 cases saw their lesions subside, and 6 cases were ineffective. At the beginning of the therapy,

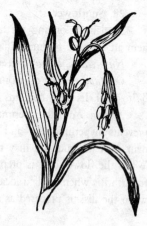

the lesions enlarged and reddened. However, persistent therapy for several more days resulted in the desquanated and withering of the lesions, which eventually dried and dropped off.

Recipe examples: (1) For rheumatism and handicapped movements of the limbs. Boil 30 g Job's-tears and 30-60 g rice to make thick porridge. Consume at a draught once daily.

(2) For pain in lower limbs with swelling, also for hemoptysis or bloody sputum. Use 50 g Job's-tears and 2 pig's trotters. Simmer with slow fire and consume the whole thing.

(3) For flat wart. Boil 40 g Job's-tears for 20 minutes. Divide into 2 equal halves and consume twice, in the morning and in the evening. Ten successive days constitute a therapeutic course.

30. Hawthorn

The fruit of a plant belonging to the rosacea family with various species.

Nature and flavour: Sweet, sour and slightly warm.

Constituents: Protein, fat, rich in vitamin C, crategolic acid, hawthorn acid, lemon acid, saponin, tannate and fructose.

Actions: Increasing secretion of digestive juices, especially beneficial for the digestion of meat. Anti-bacterial, softening the blood vessels and lowering blood pressure and blood cholesterol. In traditional Chinese medicine, it is held that it cures dyspepsia and emaciation in children, and eliminates vomiting, pain and diarrhoea.

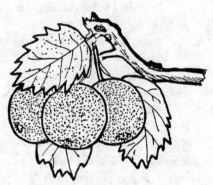

Experimental results: In animal experiments, the alcohol extracts of hawthorn slices reveal slow yet sustained drop of blood pressure. This might be due to the relaxation of blood vessels. It also stimulated the contraction of animal uterus.

Clinical reports: Forty cases of tapeworm infection were treated by hawthorn fruit administered by eating 1,000 g fresh hawthorn (or 250 g dry hawthorn) with stones discarded. The therapy began from 3 p.m. and

133

completed at 10 p.m. The cases fasted for dinner. On the next morning, each drank 1 cup of areca nut solution. All the cases were cured.

It was also reported that hawthorn was also good at lowering serum cholesterol. Boil 50 g hawthorn and 100 g Radix Ilicis Pubescentis in 200 ml water until half volume was gone. Divide the solution into 2 equal portions. After treatment, 20 cases had their blood cholesterol lowered from 253.2 mg% to 207 mg%, a drop of 46.2 mg% on average.

Recipe examples: (1) For dyspepsia due to excess ingestion of animal meat. Boil 10 g hawthorn charcoal and some brown sugar, and drink.

(2) For hypertension. Decoct 6 g hawthorn with some rock sugar and drink the decoction at a draught.

(3) For hypercholesterolemia and coronary heart disease. Boil 12 g hawthorn and half sheet of lotus leaf. Drink the solution as one would tea.

(4) For viral hepatitis. 3 g hawthorn powder and some sugar dissolved in warm water, three times daily for a course of 10 days. Several courses may be administered.

31. Sesame

Belonging to the pedaliacea family. There are two kinds of sesame, black and white.

Nature and flavour: Sweet and moderate.

Constituents: It contains much fat, mainly glyceride of oleic acid and loneleic acid, sucrose, lecithin, protein, sesamine, sesamol, sesamolin, etc. Also vitamins A, D and E.

Actions: In traditional Chinese medicine, it is claimed that sesame benefits the body as a whole, especially the spleen and stomach. Its high oil content lubricates the intestine and nourishes all the internal viscera. It also blackens one's hair, especially the black sesame. Hence, it is applied to white hair, habitual constipation, and insufficient lactation. Sesame oil is also helpful in treating intestinal worms like ascaris, tapeworm, etc.

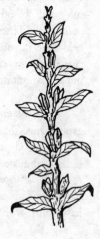

Recipe examples: (1) For general weakness and infirmity. Use 30 g black sesame and boil with 100 g glutinous rice to make porridge. Add appropriate sugar after well done.

(2) For dizziness due to deficient liver and kidney, and premature white hair. Decoct black sesame, fruit of Chinese wolfberry and tuber of multiflower knotweed, each 15 g, and 9 g chrysanthemum in water for 15 minutes under slow fire. Drink the decoction once daily for a long period of 1-2 months.

(3) For constipation, vertigo and dizziness due to deficient liver and kidney. Crush some walnut, and pulverize dry mulberry together with equal amount of black sesame. Mix all ingredients with bee honey. Administer 2-3 teaspoonfuls, 3 times daily.

(4) For chronic rhinitis with running nose. Heat 20 ml. sesame oil. Drop a few drops of cooled boiled oil to each nostril, thrice daily.

(5) For toothache. Boil 50 g sesame in 500 ml water. Use the solution for gargling.

(6) For promoting lactation. Bake sesame to brown and grind into powder. Eat as one likes.

32. Eggplant

A plant belonging to the solanacea family. There are many kinds of eggplant, elongated and oval shape, white and purplish skin, etc.

Nature and flavour: Sweet and cold.

Constituents: It contains trigonelline, stachydrine, choline, solanine, vitamins P, B and C, nicotinic acid, carotene, protein and fat.

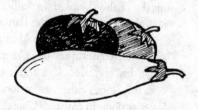

Actions: Due to its cool nature, it yields some antipyretic action. It also possesses analgesic, detumescent action and may be applied topically for ulcera. A report mentioned that the dry leaves of eggplant with purple-flower, when prepared as paste, yielded very satisfactory results (though not radical) for necrotic tissues of ulcers in cancer of mammary gland. It is also used for all kinds of bleeding, especially bloody stool and urine.

Recipe examples: (1) For bloody stool. Collect some frosted eggplant with its base intact. Bake it to scorch and prepare as powder. Administer 6 g on empty stomach, 2-3 times a day.

(2) For icteric hepatitis. Use 1,000 g eggplant with purplish skin and

decoct with rice to make porridge. Eat the porridge for several days.

(3) For chronic dysentery. Wrap 3 large eggplants with moistened paper and cover inside very hot earth until it is done. Put the hot eggplant into 1 liter of alcohol and seal the container tightly. After 3 whole days, drink the liquor in warm condition each day.

33. Calabash

A plant belonging to the cucurbitacea family. The species with the narrow-waisted fruit is applied for medicinal use.

Nature and flavour: Sweet and moderate.

Constituents: The medicinal part contains glucose, pentosan, lignin and shikimic acid. White raw fruit contains carrotene and some vitamins.

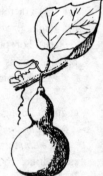

Action: It is mainly applied as a diuretic and a remedy for dribbling urination. In animal experiments, with gastric infusion of calabash decoction at a dosage of 2g/kg in rabbit, with the amount of urine markedly increased the first 12 hours. Some species of calabash contains cucurbitacin B which is toxic and may cause death in animals when injected intravenously with 0.3 mg/kg of this chemical. In traditional Chinese medicine, it is also applied in edema, flatulence and jaundice.

Remarks: Calabash is cold in nature. So people with a physical constitution of cold nature should not consume this vegetable. It is interesting to note that calabash is mostly applied as a medicine rather as a food for treating edema. It is also used in hypertension. In ancient China, the folk doctors used to hang up a dry calabash fruit outside their dispensaries as a symbol due to its special and attractive appearance. Even the traditional doctors and others in the medical sector used it as a professional symbol.

34. White gourd (wax gourd)

A plant belonging to the cucurbitacea family. Its skin and seeds are used for medicinal purposes. The flesh is also used.

Nature and flavour: Sweet and slightly cold.

Constituents: Mostly water, with some sugar, protein, cellulose, carrotene, vitamins B_1, B_2 and C, nicotinic acids, calcium, phosphorus and iron. It also contains asparagine in its flower.

Actions: This gourd is a very popular food in summer. It yields prominent diuretic action and is extensively applied in all kinds of edema of all causes, including nephritic, cardiac or hepatic illness. In thirsty disorders such as deficiency of *yin*, diabetes, summer heat and phlegm diseases, wax gourd, mostly its seeds and skin, are extensively used.

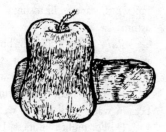

Recipe examples: (1) For chronic nephritis. Prepare a carp fish as usual. Cook it in water with 1,000 g wax gourd and consume everything.

(2) For scanty urine in pregnant woman. Use a cup of juice from white gourd mixed with some bee honey. Administer twice a day for several days.

(3) For beauty purposes. Prepare 50 g wax gourd seeds, 40 g peach flower, 20 g poplar bark. Grind together as powder. Use 5 g after meal, 3 times a day. In case poplar bark is not available, tangerine peel may be used as a substitute.

(4) For thirst in febrile disease and summer heat. Decoct 20 g inner loose part of the gourd and drink it as one would tea.

35. Pumpkin

A plant belonging to the cucurbitacea family.

Nature and flavour: Sweet and cold.

Constituents: It contains trigonelline, adenine, carrotene, vitamins B and C, glucose and sucrose. The seeds contain fat, protein, vitamins A, B_1, B_2 and C, and carrotene.

Actions: Its flesh is beneficial to body energy. The whole fruit is an anthelminthic, with raw flesh for ascaris, seeds for tapeworm. A group of 10 cases each ate up to 500 g raw flesh (250 g for children). The worms in 6 cases were expelled from the intestine. The largest number of

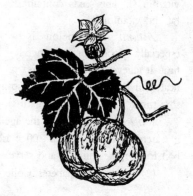

worms totalled 100; the least, 2. The seeds are powerful vermicide for ascaris, tapeworm, and schistosoma. They also relieve short breath in bronchial asthma.

Recipe examples: (1) For bronchial asthma. Steam 500 g pumpkin and then mix with some honey or sugar. Most cases can have their symptoms controlled.

(2) For bloody and purulent phlegm. Cook 500 g pumpkin and 250 g beef in water until beef is well done. Apply once daily for several days.

(3) For night blindness. Use several pumpkin flowers and cook with 200 g pig's liver. Add salt and flavouring and serve as a side dish.

(4) For habitual miscarriage. Use several base parts of the pumpkin fruit. Bake it as charcoal and pulverize. Beginning from the second month of pregnancy, use one base part and swallow it with warm boiled water.

(5) For burns. Brush pumpkin and squeeze out the juice for local application.

36. Watermelon

The fruit of a plant belonging to the cucurbitacea family. It is good for overcoming summer heat.

Nature and flavour: Sweet and cold.

Constituents: The flesh contains phosphoric acid, malic acid, fructose, glucose, amino acid, lycopene, carrotene and vitamin C. The seeds contain fat and vitamin B_2.

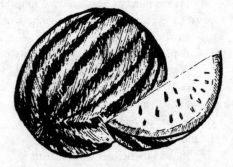

Actions: Watermelon is especially good for summer heat. It relieves thirst and clears heat, and is a good diuretic. Also applied for alcoholism. It is indicated for sore throat and aphtha (stomatitis).

Recipe examples: (1) For the aged with weak spleen function. Prepare 500 g watermelon pulp. Cook 100 g rice to make porridge. Add the pulp and boil for 2 more minutes and serve.

(2) For thirst in diabetes. Collect peels from water melon and wax gourd,

each 30 g. Decoct for 15 minutes and drink after cooled down.

(3) For dizziness and vomiting due to sun stroke. Squeeze watermelon pulp to obtain 500 ml juice. Drink 50-100 ml each time from time to time.

(4) For edema due to cardiac or nephritic diseases. Collect 60 g watermelon pulp, and 60 g cogong root. Decoct together for 10 minutes and drink as one would tea.

(5) For dyspepsia and loss of appetite. Collect juice from watermelon and tomato. Mix together and serve as tea.

37. Dark plum

The fruit of a plant belonging to the rosacea family. Made by smoking unripe green plum.

Nature and flavour: Sour and moderate.

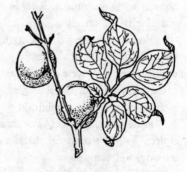

Constituents: It contains malic acid, citric acid, succinic acid, ß-sitosterol, triterpene, etc.

Actions: Marked anti-bacterical action, especially to bacillus E coli, dysentery, typhoid fever, cholera bacilli and Pseudo-monas aeruginosa. In traditional Chinese medicine, it is an antipyretic, antiascaris remedy with astringent action.

Experiment results: When water solution made of dark plum (1:1) was researched in laboratory, it was found that the solution inhibited many kinds of bacteria except streptococcus A and B. It also yielded anti-fungus action in vitro to a dilution of 1:480. Moreover, its solution also presented guinea pig form anaphylactic alock due to some allergin.

Recipe example: (1) For protracted coughing. Grind equal amount of plum flesh slightly backed with honey-fried poppyshell as powder. Swallow with diluted honey water before going to bed, once daily.

(2) For bloody and purulent diarrhoea. Use stoned dark plum, 30 g. Bake and prepare as powder. Administer 6 g and swallow with porridge soup.

(3) For thirst due to fever. Boil 2-5 pieces of dark plum in water and add 50-100 g sugar and then drink.

Remarks: Do not consume too much plum or it may cause some emotional disturbances.

38. Chinese dates (including wild jujube)

There are many kinds of dates in China, including red, black and wild jujube, all belonging to the rhamnacea family. Black dates are processed first by drying red dates under sunlight, and then steaming and baking. After repeating the process several times, black dates are obtained.

Nature and flavour: Red dates are sweet and moderate, wild jujube sour and moderate.

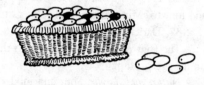

Constituents: Protein, sugar, organic acid, and mucus. Rich in vitamins B_2, C, and P.

Actions: Chinese dates are tonics for the spleen and stomach and nourish the body fluids. They also reveal some sedative effect. In animal experiments, when rabbits were poisoned with CCl_4, with ensuing liv r functional impairment, they were protected by a solution of dates, resulting in an increase of blood albumin.

Recipe examples: (1) For weak digestive function, including pept c ulcer. Use 10 stoned red dates, and 50 g glutinous rice for porridge. After cooking, add some sugar.

(2) For anemia. Prepare a sheep's vertebral column, 20 stoned Chinese red dates, 50-100 g glutinous rice. Cook together to make porridge. After cooking, add salt and flavourings. Consume in 2-3 parts within a single day.

(3) For purpura. Cook 10-15 Chinese red dates. After boiling for 15 minutes, consume the whole solution with date stones discarded, three times a day.

39. Pear

The fruit of a plant belonging to the rosacea family, including various species. For medicinal use, those with thin skin, tender and juicy flesh are preferable.

Nature and flavour: Sweet and cold.

Constituents: Containing malic acid, glucose, sucrose, vitamins B and C.

Actions: Since pear is cold in nature and juicy, it is a moistening agent and produces fluids in the body. It used to be applied in febrile diseases for thirst, constipation and diabetes.

Recipe examples: (1) For feverish diseases with thirsty mouth and throat. Use a large fresh pear. Cut it into thin slices. Soak it in cold boiled water for half a day. Squeeze to obtain juice. Drink it bit by bit as you like.

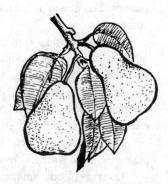

(2) For high fever. Cut 3 large pears into slices. Boil in 3,000 ml water with slow fire until half the water volume is gone. Discard the residue. Add 50 g rice to make porridge.

(3) For short breath and coughing with phlegm. Peel 1-2 pears with the seeds eliminated. Cut into pieces. Add 10 pieces of almond and 20 g rock sugar. Steam in 200 ml water for 30 minutes. Drink it all at a draught.

40. Persimmon

The fruit of a plant belonging to the ebenacea family. Both fresh and dried persimmon (called persimmon cake in China) are used for medicinal purposes.

Nature and flavour: Sweet and cold. The white powder on the surface of dried persimmon is sweet and moderate, while the calyx is puckery.

Constituents: Containing sucrose, glucose, fructose and iodine. The calyx contains triterpene, olive acid and ursolic acid. Powder of dried persimmon contains manitole, glucose, fructose, sucrose and vitamin C.

Actions: The astragalin extracted from persimmon leaves lowers blood pressure and increases blood flow in coronary arteries. In TCM, it is claimed that persimmon is an antipyretic, while its dry white powder moistens the lungs and heart. The calyx is good for

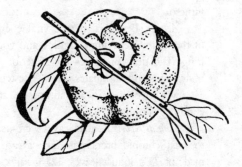

hiccups. Persimmon is capable of lowering blood pressure and is good for constipation.

Clinical report: In a group of 194 cases of chronic bronchitis, acupoint injection of persimmon extract in water solution (0.3 g persimmon/g) was administered, 0.3-0.5 ml each point, once daily or every other day. Results revealed that 71 cases (36.5 percent) were clinically controlled, 66 cases (34 percent) markedly effective, 51 cases (26.2 percent) ameliorated and only 6 cases ineffective. The total effective rate: 96.7 percent.

Recipe examples: (1) For bloody urine. Cut persimmon cakes into small pieces and cook with glutinous rice to make porridge. Administer each day.

(2) For bloody sputum (hemoptysis). Bake 3 persimmon cakes to charcoal, and grind into powder. Dissolve 6 g in water and drink at a draught, three times a day.

(3) For hypertension. Use a green (immature) persimmon. Obtain its juice and drink three times a day. Or use 10 persimmon cakes for decoction.

(4) For cold and water diarrhoea. Steam 2 persimmon cakes over steaned rice and eat it at one sitting.

41. Loquat

A plant belonging to the rosacea family. The fruit, kernel and tender leaves are all used for medicinal purposes.

Nature and flavour: Sweet, sour and moderate.

Constituents: Its flesh contains malic acid, tartaric acid, citric acid, tannate, carrotene, vitamins A, B and C. Its leaves and kernel contain amygdalin, nerolidol and farnesol.

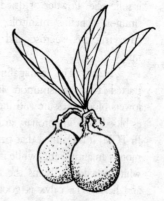

Actions: Beneficial to the vital energy of the lungs. Relieving coughing and vomiting. The flesh promotes the secretion of body fluids and eliminates thirst. The tender leaves, free of hair, are antitussive and eliminate sputum.

Clinical report: Loquat leaves were used to treat chronic bronchitis. The syrup is made of 75 g loquat leaves, 125 g calyx of eggplant boiled in 3,000 ml water until

2,000 ml remain. Add sugar to make 240 ml syrup. Administer 10 ml, 3 times a day, with 20 days constituted as a therapeutic course. In a group of 167 cases, 42 (25 percent) were clinically controlled, 60 (36 percent) markedly effective, 35 (20 percent) ameliorated, with only 30 (18 percent) ineffective.

Recipe examples: (1) For difficult urination, dry throat. Consume 250 g fresh loquat flesh (pulp) in two equal parts, in morning and evening.

(2) For chronic coughing. Pound 15 g loquat seed and then boil in water with 3 thin slices of ginger. Drink 50 ml of the solution, 2-3 times a day. A little honey may also be mixed.

(3) Decoct 20 g dry loquat leaves for 15 minutes. Drink the solution as one would tea.

42. Tangerine

The fruit of a plant belonging to the rutacea family. The species vary. Besides its flesh, the skin and pith are also used for medicinal purposes.

Nature and flavour: Flesh (sweet, sour and warm). Skin (pungent and warm).

Constituents: In its skin are hesperidin, citric acid, malic acid, glucose, sucrose, vitamin C; the flesh contains carotene, vitamin C (a little less than in the skin), cryptoxanthin, vitamin B_1. The ingredients in the skin also contain volatile oil, mainly limonene. Some species also contain isopropenyltoluene, etc.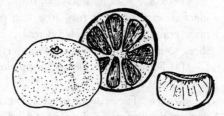

Actions: In addition to the flesh, which possesses the actions of stimulating appetite, regulating *qi* circulation and producing fluids to moisten the lung, the peel is an even more useful medicinal food. Extracts from tangerine peel strengthens the contraction of cardiac muscle to increase its blood output of toad heart in vitro. The hesperidin, in animal experiments, is antagonistic to adrenalin that constricts the blood vessels. It also strengthens the contraction of involuntary muscles in the intestine. Moreover, hesperidin also reveals some antiphlogistic, cholegogic actions. Hence, tangerine peels are extensively applied for strengthening the spleen-stomach (digestion), regulating *qi* circulation to stop nausea and vomiting, also as an antitussive and expectorant.

Clinical reports: An old friend of mine was a heavy smoker. He used to suffer bronchitis attacks with itching throat, profuse phlegm secretion and a poor appetite. I advised him to take an old traditional ready-made bolus, containing tangerine peel as major ingredient, and make great efforts to reduce his smoking, if not quit totally. He agreed, taking the bolus for one month and reducing his smoking to as much as only one half the original quantity. He told me 2 months later that his condition had mitigated very much. But itching throat and mild coughing still existed. I further advised him and gave a modified prescription, i.e., using processed tangerine peel as a substitute for tea and as a routine beverage. He was nearly cured a year later, though not totally. This, I think, should be attributed to the merit of tangerine peel and his smoking habit should be the only cause for his not being entirely free from coughing.

Recipe example: (1) For vomiting, coughing with profuse sputum. Decoct 10 g tangerine peel, 3 g ginger in 150 ml water for 15 minutes and add some brown sugar. Drink at a draught.

(2) For dyspepsia and anorexia. Soak 50 g tangerine peel in 500 ml liquor for 7 days. Drink a small cup each day.

(3) For epigastric distention, belching. Collect 9 g tangerine peel, 12 g inner skeleton of cuttle fish, 50 g lean pork. Cook these with 50 g rice to make porridge. After porridge is ready, discard the peel and bone. Add pork slices, some salt and flavourings, and serve.

(4) For poor digestion and dissipating sputum. Use 30 g tangerine peel as a substitute for tea.

Remarks: The network structure on the inner wall of tangerine peel and that on the surface of the flesh (called tangerine reticulum) is even more effective for expectoration, coughing and improving *qi* flow.

43. Banana

The fruit of a plant belonging to the musacea family.

Nature and flavour: Sweet and cold.

Constituents: It contains starch, protein, fat, vitamins A, B, C and E and a little nor-adrenaline and serotinin dopamine.

Actions: Banana is good at nourishing *yin* principle of the body, lubricates the intestine and facilitates bowel movements. It also has some detoxifying and antipyretic effect. Hence, it is indicated in febrile diseases when constipation, thirst and restlessness occur. It is also helpful in tackling hemorrhoids.

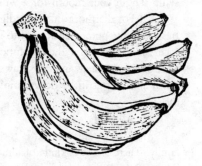

Recipe examples: (1) For protracted coughing with constipation. Use 2 peeled bananas and boil with some rock sugar. Consume 1-2 times a day for several successive days.

(2) For hemorrhoids with blood stool. Cook 2 unpeeled bananas. After 10 minutes, consume the cooled down fruit with peel. Half-ripe ones are preferable.

(3) For hypertension with constipation. Difficulty in defecation may be troublesome to hypertensive patients, especially the elderly. It may even cause serious accidents such as stroke. Normal bowel movements are vital to their health. Use 500 g peeled banana and mix with 15 g black sesame to form a mixture. Divide into 2 equal halves. Administer twice daily.

(4) For asthma and short breath. The recipe is basically similar to that of No. 2 for hemorrhoids. But this time the unpeeled bananas should be very soft or a little bit over-mature.

44. Pomegranate

The fruit of a plant belonging to the punicacea family. The skin is used for medicinal purposes. Sometimes its root and flower are also used.

Nature and flavour: Sweet, pungent, sour and warm.

Constituents: The fruit skin contains tannic acid, resin, gallic acid, innositol, sugar and gum. The skin of its root contains isopelletierine.

Actions: The skin of its root is an anthelminthic. Pomegranate skin reveals strong inhibition to typhoid bacilli. In TCM, it is an astringent.

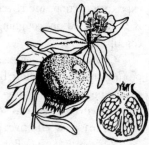

Recipe examples: (1) For stomatitis. Pound pomegranate seeds to obtain its juice to which a little sugar or rock candy is added. Drink the juice as you like. Let the syrup stay in your mouth for a while before swallowing.

(2) For diarrhoea due to indigestion and enteritic abdominal pain. Use fresh or white pomegranate peel to make decoction. Boil twice and separately, each 30 minutes. Mix the 2 solutions and concentrate it by slow fire. Then add some bee honey and move away from the fire once it boils again. Cool down and keep it in bottle. Administer 2 times a day with 1 teaspoonful for each dose.

45. Almond

Almond, or apricot nut, is the fruit of a plant belonging to the rosacea family. There are two kinds of almond, bitter and sweet. The bitter almond is mostly applied for medicinal purpose.

Nature and flavour: The whole apricot fruit is sour, sweet and warm; the nut is bitter and warm, with little toxicity.

Constituents: The apricot fruit contains malic acid, vitamin C, carrotene, and volatile oil in which myr-cene, limonene, terpenolene, gera-niol, linalool and neral are in-cluded. In the almond, there are emulsin, amygdalin and fat-ty acids.

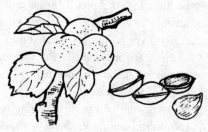

Actions: Three percent of amygdalin is contained in bitter almond. This amygdalin can be decomposed by amygdalinase into mandelonitrile and prunasin which, under suitable condition, may be further hydrolyzed into cyanic acid. Trace amount of cyanic acid yields antitussive and expectorant action. Moreover, it also has some lubricating action. So, almond is always used in coughing due to various kinds of causes, as well as constipation.

Clinical reports: 124 cases of chronic bronchitis, manifesting coughing, profuse sputum and short breath were treated with almond candy, made of equal amount (9 g) of bitter almond and rock sugar, twice a day for 10 days. The total effective rate was 96.8 percent in which 23 cases were basically cured, 66 cases markedly effective, and 31 ameliorated.

Recipe examples: (1) For short breath and edema. Fry 30 g almond with its skin and tips eliminated. Cook with rice to make porridge, and eat on empty stomach.

(2) For chronic coughing due to deficient lungs and kidneys. Boil 250 g fried almond for 1 hour. Then add 250 g walnut and continue to boil until the water evaporates totally. Add 500 g honey and stir thoroughly. Eat 1-2 teaspoonfuls, twice a day.

Remarks: Since cyanic acid is extremely toxic, extreme care should be given to over consumption. It is estimated that the lethal dosage for an adult is 0.05 g: for a little child, 7-10 pieces of bitter almond are enough to produce lethal intoxication.

46. Papaya

The fruit of a plant belonging to the caricacea family.

Nature and flavour: Sweet and cold.

Constituents: Containing carpaine, papain, cryptoxanthine, rennin, violaxanthin, carrotene and lycopene.

Actions: It promotes digestion with some bacteriostatic action and also stimulates bowel movements, so it may be tried for dysentery and constipation. Besides, there are some reports demonstrating its anti-tumour action.

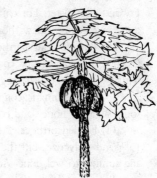

Recipe examples: (1) For thirst and chronic coughing. Use 250-500 g ripe fresh papaya and steam. Eat twice a day.

(2) For indigestion and abdominal pain. Use 500 g green unripe papaya. Remove its peel and seeds and cut into cubes in the size of walnut. Soak in vinegar for 2-3 days. Eat 30 g twice daily.

(3) For intestinal parasites. Use 50 ml vinegar prepared from the above recipe at bedtime.

(4) For boils and carbuncles. Smash 250 g ripe fresh papaya and apply locally.

47. Gingko

Commonly called "silver apricot," it belong to the ginkgoasea family. Its fruit is used for medicinal purposes.

Nature and flavour: Sweet, bitter, puckery and toxic.

Constituents: Containing ginkgolic acid, bilobol, ginnol, gibberellin, sugar, tannate, fatty oil, starch and protein.

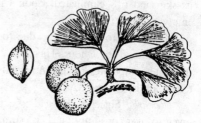

Actions: It is basically astringent in nature and is therefore applied for asthmatic coughing, leucorrhea and bed-wetting. In traditional Chinese medicine, it is also applied in pulmonary tuberculosis.

Clinical reports: Experimental therapy was made clinically in pulmonary tuberculosis, treated by gingko soaked in raw vegetarian oil. Though it relieves symptoms to some extent, no radical cure has been reported.

Recipe examples: (1) For bed-wetting. Crush the shell and obtain the nuts. Fry and administer. For children under 10, 5-7 nuts; for adults, less than 10 nuts, twice daily. Chew thoroughly.

(2) For infantile diarrhoea. Prepare 4 gingko nuts and grind as powder. Open small hole at one end of an egg and fill the hole with powder. Seal with paper and boil the egg until it is done. Consume the whole egg.

(3) For asthmatic coughing. Shell 10 gingkos and boil in water. Add some sugar or honey and consume.

(4) For leucorrhoea. Prepare gingko nut, lotus seed, glutinous rice, each 15 g and pulverize. Fill the powder inside the cavity of black-bone chicken and simmer to wel done. Add salt and flavourings and serve.

Remarks: Gingko is somewhat poisonous and too much should not be eaten. In traditional Chinese medicine, no more than 10 nuts can be eaten at one time. Special care should be taken to keep children from over eating. Manifestations of poisoning include vomiting, fever or even convulsion.

48. Walnut

The fruit of a plant belonging to the jugladacea family. Its nuts are applied for medicinal use.

Nature and flavour: Sweet and warm.

Constituents: Containing much fat mainly linoleic acid, also protein, vitamins B_1 and B_2, tannate, citrulline and juglone.

Actions: The fat in walnut is beneficial to the formation of albumin in the body. In TCM, it is claimed that walnut is warm yet not dry like most nuts; hence, it is good for weakness and deficient vital essence in the elderly, nourishing the blood and vital energy, benefitting the lungs and kidneys and moistening the lungs.

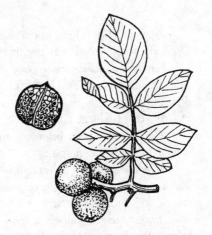

Clinical reports: It has been reported that walnut is effective for urinary infections and stones. Moreover, many kinds of dermatitis without secondary infection and eczema were reported to have been satisfactorily cured by walnut zinc oxide paste applied 1-2 times daily. Most cases were cured within 1-10 days.

Recipe examples: (1) For asthma of deficient type. Pound 1,000 g walnut and mix with 500 ml bee honey. Administer 1-2 teaspoonfuls each day.

(2) For nausea and acid regurgitation. Crush several walnuts and swallow with ginger solution.

(3) For habitual constipation. Prepare 20 g walnut and 20 g black sesame, all fried to a little bit brown. Eat at bedtime once daily.

(4) For urine dribbling, insomnia and forgetfulness. Crush 50 g walnut, and consume as one likes.

49. Mulberry fruit

The fruit of a plant belonging to the moracea family.

Nature and flavour: Sweet and moderate.

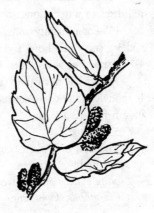

Constituents: Rich in carotene, vitamins B_1, B_2 and C, glucose, sucrose, tartaric acid and succinic acid.

Actions: Benefitting vital energy and eliminating excessive fluids.

149

Recipe examples: (1) For insomnia. Decoct 30-50 g mulberry fruit in water. Drink the whole solution at one draught before bedtime.

(2) For rheumatic pain in body. Prepare 200 g mulberry fruit. Boil under slow fire until pasty. Divide the paste in 3 equal parts, and consume in 3 dosages.

50. Dried longan pulp

The fruit of a plant belonging to the sapindacea family. The dried fruit is used for medicinal purposes.

Nature and flavour: Sweet and warm.

Constituents: Rich in glucose, sucrose, choline and vitamins B and C, tartaric acid, protein and fat.

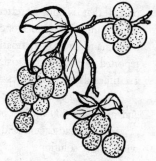

Actions: Longan pulp is a tonic for the spleen, the heart and blood. In traditional Chinese conception, it benefits the heart and promotes one's intelligence. It is used to check palpitation, insomnia and dreamy sleep due to over-anxiousness; loss of appetite, general malaise, and watery diarrhoea due to hypofunction of the spleen. It is especially good for postpartum anemia.

Recipe examples: (1) For anemia. Use 5 g dry longan pulp, 10 g lotus seeds and 100 g rice to cook porridge at meal.

(2) For dizziness, general weakness. Cook 30 g dry longan pulp, 30 g red dates in water. Consume at a draught.

(3) For infirmity and postpartum weakness. Put 30 g dry longan pulp and 3 g sugar in a bowl and then cover with gauze. Steam and then consume 1-2 teaspoonful with boiled water.

Remarks: Longan pulp, either dry or fresh, is believed to be quite warm. It is advisable not to take too much longan, or epistaxis and dry throat and mouth may result.

51. Grape

The fruit of a plant belonging to the vitacea family. It is, together with its wine, highly nutritious.

Nature and flavour: Sweet and moderate.

Constituents: Containing polysaccharides, especially rich in glucose and sucrose. Also contain protein, carrotene, vitamins B₁, B₂ and C.

Actions: Grape is a tonic for both *qi* and blood. It strengthens one's tendons and bones, and yields diuretic action. It is indicated in deficient *qi* and blood, good at stopping coughing due to *yin* deficiency, manifesting palpitation, night sweats and rheumatism.

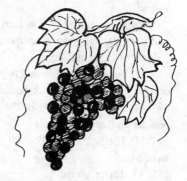

Recipe examples: (1) For anemia and sour pain in the knee and waist due to kidney deficiency. Prepare wine made by fermenting grape juice. Apply 10-20 ml twice a day.

(2) For bacillary dysentery. Pound rinsed fresh grape and ginger, 500 g and 200 g, respectively. Wrap with clean gauze to obtain juice separately. Boil concentrated green tea. To each cup add 50 ml grape juice and 20 ml ginger juice. Add a little honey and drink hot.

(3) For thirst in febrile disease. Obtain some grape juice. Boil and concentrate the juice to form sticky jelly. Add a little bee honey to form paste. Add a teaspoonful of the paste to a cup of water and drink.

(4) For bloody urine. Crush 120 g fresh grapes and 280 g fresh lotus roots. Obtain juice from both and consume the juice. This may be repeated 3 times a day.

52. Guava

The fruit of a plant belonging to the myrtacea family.

Nature and flavour: Sweet and moderate.

Constituents: The fruit contains ß-sitosterol, guaijaverin, gallic acid, vitamin C, sugars and quercetin.

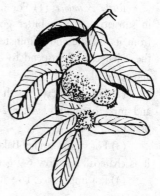

Actions: In TCM, it is claimed that guava stops diarrhoea and bleeding, with antiphlogistic, astringent and drying actions. The fruit juice is a remedy for diabetes mellitus. The green and immature fruit, after having been baked and ground into powder, is good for wounds.

Recipe examples: (1) For acute dysentery. Smash 250 g fresh guava and boil it in 500 ml water to evaporate half its volume. Divide into 3 parts for 3 doses to be administered in a day. Repeat for several days until cured.

(2) For diabetes. Crush 250 g fresh guava and obtain the juice which is divided into 3 doses. Drink one dose each time, 3 times a day.

(3) For wounds. Crush 250 g fresh guava and bake it dry. Grind into powder and apply topically.

(4) For hoarseness. Boil 90 g dry guava in 200 ml water. Serve as one would tea.

53. Bitter gourd
A plant belonging to the cucurbitacea family.

Nature and flavour: Bitter and cold.

Constituents: Containing charantin, 5-hydroxytryptamine, vitamin C, some amino acids etc.

Actions: It is claimed, in TCM, that this gourd clears the evil fire of the heart and improves eyesight, while its fruit strengthens the vital energy and sexual power. It also relieves thirst, sunstroke and carbuncles.

Recipe examples: (1) For fever in sunstroke. Cut a bitter gourd from its middle and eliminate its pulp. Fill its cavity with green tea. Unite the 2 halves and suspend to dry in the shadow. Then boil 6-9 g each time and serve like tea.

(2) For dysentery. Smash a bitter gourd to make paste. Add 100 g sugar and mix thoroughly. After 2 hours, squeeze out the juice and drink at a draught.

(3) For stomachache. Bake a bitter gourd brown until scorched and grind it as charcoal. Swallow 6-9 g with water whenever needed.

(4) For impotence. Use 50 g seeds from bitter gourd and bake dry. Grind

into powder. Use 6-9 g each time, swallow with boiled water.

54. Carambola

The fruit of a plant belonging to the cucurbitacea family.

Nature and flavour: Sweet, slightly puckery and moderate.

Constituents: Containing sugar, vitamins B₁, B₂ and C, malic acid and citric acid.

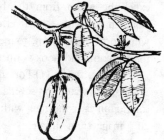

Actions: Increasing the formation of body fluids, acting as an antitussive, and beneficial to digestion.

Recipe examples: (1) For redness of urine, pain and dribbling. Consume 2 fresh mature carambolas at a draught. Repeat twice daily.

(2) For flaring up of inner fire with toothache, red eyes, stomatitis and sore throat. Crush 3 carambolas and then squeeze to obtain juice. Drink all the juice. Repeat 2-3 times a day.

(3) For difficult urination. Crush 3 mature fresh carambolas, and obtain juice. Drink all the juice. Repeat the process 2-3 times when necessary.

55. Betel nut

The fruit of a plant belonging to the palma family.

Nature and flavour: Warm and pungent.

Constituents: Containing much alkaloid, tannate, fat and areca red, with arecaline as its main constituent. Other alkaloids include arecaine, quvacine, etc.

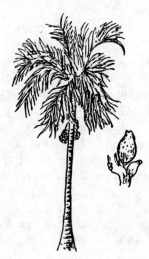

Actions: Betal nut reveals anthelminthic action and is mainly applied for tapeworm and ascaris. But it is ineffective for schistosoma. The arecoline can increase saliva secretion, intestinal peristalsis, lower heart rate and blood pressure and constrict bronchial muscles in animal experiments. It also improves digestive function and memory.

Clinical reports: It has been reported that betal nut was administered as anthelminthes. When combining with pumpkin seeds, about three dozen cases were reported to have an effective rate of 90-95 percent.

It was claimed that the arecoline in betel nut only paralyzes the tapeworm, but doesn't expel it from the intestine. So, cathartic is needed to expel the worm from the body. Moreover, betel nut is also applied in clonorchiasis with a total effective rate of 47.2-90 percent. Also good for whipworm, hookworm, roundworm and pinworm, but it is not satisfactory for pinworm and hookworm. For whipworm, it is rather satisfactory.

Recipe examples: (1) For tapeworm. Use 60-100 g betel nut and soak with 300-500 ml water for several hours. Then boil to half volume. Drink the solution in early morning with empty stomach. About 1 hour later, administer 20 g magnesium sulfate.

(2) For abdominal flatulence. Boil 15 g betel nut with 50 g pork for 15 minutes, and consume the soup with pork together.

Remarks: People with a history of coronary heart disease are banned from ingesting betel nut.

56. Cucumber

The fruit of plant belonging to the cucurbitacea family. It can be served raw.

Nature and flavour: Sweet and cold.

Constituents: Containing sugar, protein, vitamin C and volatile oil, free amino acids, rutin, and chlorogenic acid. Its base is slightly bitter containing cucurbitacin A, B, C and D.

Actions: It clears fever, facilitates water excretion and has antitoxic effect. It is mainly applied for flaring up of evil fire, such as sore throat, red eyes and thirst.

Recipe examples: (1) For hot diarrhoea in children. Use a tender cucumber. After thorough rinsing, eat raw after tossing it with bee honey.

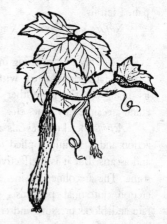

(2) For edema. Use 50 g old cucumber and boil in water twice daily. It is good for mild edema of the extremities.

(3) For digestive type common cold with diarrhoea, low fever and abdominal pain. Use several fresh cucumber leaves. Boil for 1 hour. Discard residue and add some sugar. Drink the solution at a draught.

D. Meat, Fowl and Seafood

1. Chicken

A fowl belonging to the phasianidae family. Almost all its body parts have medicinal uses. However, chicken meat, the inner layer of the gizzard, eggs and egg shell are the most commonly used.

Nature and flavour: Flesh, sweet and warm; and egg, sweet and moderate.

Constituents: Chicken meat is rich in protein, fat, minerals, including calcium, potassium, sodium and iron, vitamins A, B_1, B_2, C and E and nicotinic acid. Its egg contains high contents of protein, fat, vitamins A, B_1 and B_2, and nicotinic acid, minerals, including calcium, phosphorus, iron. It also contains ovalbumin, ovomucoid, ovomucin, and conalbumin. In the yolk, it contains lecithin, fatty acids and lutein. The gizzard contains ventriculin. The shell contains mainly calcium carbonate, calcium phosphate, magnesium phosphate, with some porphyrin.

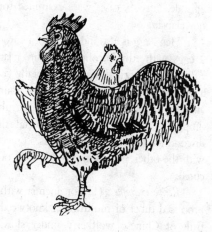

Actions: Chicken is not only delicious, but also therapeutically very effective. In traditional Chinese medicine, it is a tonic with warm nature and beneficial to blood and *qi*, nourishing the essence and spirit. An old hen is even more nutritious for the infirm, pregnant women and the aged. It also invigorates the function of the spleen and stomach.

The egg as a whole is again a very strong tonic. It nourishes the blood and *yin* principle and protects the foetus. For those cases at the convalescent stage of diseases, such as febrile disease, anemia, *yin* deficiency, wounds and consumption disorders, hen's egg is the most ideal nutrient due not only to its high nutritious contents, but also to its digestibility. Egg shell, when used in powder form, is good at stopping epigastric pain, rickets in children and osteomalacia in adults. The inner membranous layer (called "phoenix cloth" in traditional pharmacology) nourishes *yin* and benefits the lung, and is applied in chronic coughing and hoarseness.

Clinical reports: It was reported that hen's egg, when boiled in bittern water, is good for malaria therapy. Boil appropriate amount of bittern (12-15 ml for adult, 3-5 ml for children younger than 5 years old, 5-8 ml for 5-9 years old, 9-11 ml for 10-18 years old). Crush 2 shells and put into the boiling bittern. Stir thoroughly until it becomes a pie. Administer immediately. Out of 66 cases thus treated, 44 were cured for escaping the coming malarial episode. Fifty-six cases were examined for follow-up. All but 3 cases revealed no relapsing.

Hen's egg is also indicated for neurodermatitis and psoriasis. First sterilize 2 eggs with ethyl alcohol. Place in a jar only slightly larger than the eggs. Add vinegar until the eggs are totally covered. Seal the jar and let stand for a week. Then break the shell and pour the egg white and egg yolk into another sterilized jar and seal. Now, rub the skin lesion with a cotton ball dipped in the prepared egg, several times a day. It is advisable not to discontinue the therapy. Nine cases out of 12 with neurodermitis were cured, with the other 3 cases improved. Two out of 5 cases with psoriasis were also cured.

Recipe examples: (1) For anemia with dizziness. Boil 250 g chicken, 15 g processed tuber of multiflower knotweed, 15 g Radix Angelica sinensis, 15 g fruit of Chinese wolfberry under slow fire until the meat is well done. Consume it in two doses.

(2) For lying-in women, the aged, the infirm and weak patients at convalescent stage. Treat an old hen as usual. Rub the clean hen with a thin layer of salt on its outer and inner surfaces. Fill the cavity with 10 pieces of mushroom, 15 g red Chinese dates (after soaked in warm water). Add some millet wine, ginger slices, white onion bulb, monosodium glutamate and 500 ml water. Steam for 2 hours and serve.

(3) For prolapse of anus, uterus with anemia, profuse sweating, sallow complexion. Prepare a hen of 1,000 g as usual and put in boiling water for 1 minute, and set aside. Rinse some root of membranous milk vetch. Cut the hen into large cubes and put in a pot with 1,000 ml water. Cut the root into 5-7 cm segments. Add ginger, Chinese onion, millet wine and salt. Cook with slow fire until well done. Discard the root residue and consume the whole thing in one or two parts.

(4) For tuberculosis with short breath, coughing and general weekness. Cook 250 g chicken with 9 g Chinese caterpillar fungus until well done. Add salt, onion and flavourings and serve.

(5) For loss of appetite and mild epigastric pain due to deficient spleen-stomach. Prepare a cock as usual. Remove all the viscera, and put in 18 g dangshen (Codonopsis Pilosula), 3 g tangerine peel, 3 g cinnamon bark, 6 g dry ginger, 10 pieces of peppermint. Add some flavourings, including onion, fresh ginger, soya bean sauce or salt, until the cock is well done. Consume at 2 meals on the same day or in 2 days.

Remarks: In China, there is a special species of rooster, the black-bone chicken. It is maintained that this chicken is far more nutritious as a tonic than the ordinary chicken, especially for the women. To identify a black-bone chicken, just examine its tongue. A black tongue also indicates it is a black-bone chicken.

2. Duck

A fowl belonging to the anatidae family.

Nature and flavour: Sweet and cold.

Constituents: Basically the same as those of chicken, with magnesium, potassium and sodium.

Actions: Though constituents of the duck are basically the same as that of chicken from a modern nutriological viewpoint, it is rather different from a traditional dietotherapeutic standpoint. This is simply because the nature of duck flesh is cold, while that of chicken is warm. Hence, the duck is far better for nourishing the *yin* principle and clearing inner heat. Moreover,

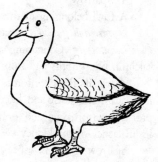

duck flesh yields some diuretic action: It is often applied in edema of various causes, such as nutritional, hepatic or nephritis.

Recipe examples: (1) For ascitis and edema. Boil a duck after treated in usual way until well done. Use a portion of the whole duck to make porridge. Prepare porridge with 100 g rice and the part of the duck as routine and serve.

(2) For *yin* deficiency manifesting night sweats, impotence, emission and weak knees and waist, etc. Prepare 10 g Chinese caterpillar fungi, a male duck, 15 ml millet wine, 5 g ginger, 10 g white bulb of Chinese onion, 5 g powdered peppermint, 3 g salt. The duck is treated as usual with inner viscera discarded and rinsed. Boil in boiling water for 1 minute. Put it with all the other ingredients in an earthenware pot. Add sufficient water and cook with slow fire for 2 hours until well done. Divide into 2 parts and serve.

(3) For sudden edema, difficult urination, fidgetiness (acute nephritis). Use 5-10 ducks' heads and clean. Smash into small pieces and mix thoroughly with some duck's blood. Add 60 g Chinese fangji (Stephania Tetrandra) and 10 g Semen Lepidii seu Descurainiae and mix again. Make pills in the size of green beans. Swallow 70 pills each time.

(4) For chronic nephritis with edema. Put 4 or 5 cloves of garlic inside a routinely prepared duck. Simmer with water until the duck is very well done. Do not add salt. Consume the whole thing.

Remarks: For weakness like hypertension with dizziness, duck is preferable. In TCM, chicken flesh is claimed as wind-type and is not suitable for patients with dizziness due to blood deficiency, while duck flesh is claimed as water-type, so it is preferable for those with deficiency of *yin*-principle and weakness of the kidney.

3. Sparrow

A fowl belonging to the ave family.

Nature and flavour: Sweet and warm.

Constituents: Containing protein, fat, calcium, phosphorus and iron.

Action: Its flesh reinforces sexual activity, warms the waist and knees, and treats profuse metrorrhagia and polyuria due to insufficiency of the kidney.

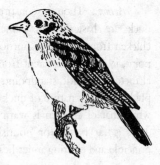

Sparrow's egg is especially good at

invigorating man's *yang* principle indicated for hyposexuality and also good at nourishing woman's blood.

Recipe examples: (1) For the infirm, aged and lack of *yang* principle. Kill several sparrows. Treat and clean as usual. Eliminate the inner viscera, except the liver. Dip into boiling water for 1 minute. Use 250 ml vegetable oil and heat to almost boiling. Oil fry sparrows until brown in colour. Then put in a pot. Add millet wine and water. Boil for 10 minutes. Place 150 g rice (or millet) to make porridge. When porridge is ready, add salt and other flavourings. Eat the porridge as one likes.

(2) For impotence and premature ejaculation. Soak 6 routinely treated sparrows in 1,000 ml millet wine, and add 20 g fruit of Chinese wolfberry. Immerse for 7 days. Drink 1-2 small cups of wine each day.

(3) For pertusis (whooping cough). Treat a sparrow as usual and simmer with 9 g rock sugar to well done. Consume once daily.

4. Cormorant

A fowl belonging to the phalacrocoracidae family. Its saliva is also a kind of medicine.

Nature and flavour: Sour and salt.

Constituents: Its flesh is rich in protein.

Actions: Cormorant's flesh is good as a diuretic. Its feathers, after burnt as ash, are good at treating fish bone stuck in the pharynx while its saliva secretion can be used for whooping cough in children.

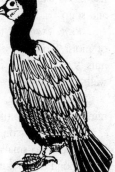

Recipe examples: (1) For ascitis. Treat a cormorant in usual way and cook in water with 60 g poria until the flesh is well done. Consume at one sitting.

(2) For fish bone in the throat. Obtain some cormorant feathers. Burn them and collect the ash. Boil 15 g tangerine peel in 100 ml water and swallow 6 g of the ash with this solution. It may be repeated several times until cured.

(3) For whooping cough. Obtain 1 ml saliva from cormorant and dissolve in boiled water. Drink at a draught.

5. Pig

An animal belonging to the suidae family. The commonest domesticated animal in China, with its meat, skin and viscerae all used for medical purposes.

Nature and flavour: Flesh, sweet and slightly cold; skin, sweet and cool; bile, bitter and cold; stomach, sweet and warm; and liver, sweet, warm and moderate.

Constituents: Lean flesh is rich in protein fat, vitamins B_1, B_2 and C; skin, rich in gelatious protein; liver, rich in iron, protein and vitamin A; bile, bilirubin; and stomach, digestive enzyme.

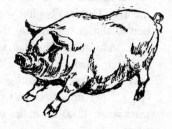

Actions: Flesh, nourishing to weakness; skin, a subsidiary remedy for hemoptysis, nasal bleeding and for regulating menstruation; liver, good for improving eyesight and as a blood tonic. For anaemia and weakness, cook flesh and liver in water with 10 g angelica sinensis. For dyspepsia, stew stomach with lotus seed and take once daily for several days. For irregular menstruation leading to anaemia, use 200 g skin simmered until sticky. Then take regularly, eating both skin and soup.

Recipe examples: (1) For dry cough with scanty sputum due to shortage of moist fluid in the lung. Use 150 g lean pork together with 9 g apricot nuts, 92 g lily, 15 g root of straight lady bell. Boil together until the pork is well done. Consume the pork and soup at one sitting.

(2) For anemia. Boil 100 g pig's liver and 50 g spinach together for 10 minutes. Consume the whole thing at one time.

(3) For dry cough with scant phlegm. Thoroughly clean a set of pig's lungs. Cut into small pieces. Add 200 g turnip, also cut as small pieces, and 9 g almond. Decoct it together in water until well done. Drink the soup and eat the lung.

(4) For hypofunction of digestion. Thoroughly clean a pig's stomach. Simmer it with 25 g Chinese yam and 100 g rice until quite well done. Consume the whole thing in 2 meals.

(5) For thirsty disorder and polyuria. Obtain a complete set of pig's pan-reas. Bake dry and prepare as powder. Swallow 3-6 g each time with warmed boiled water.

Note: For hypertension and overweight patients, do not take too much pork, especially lard and viscerae. Patients with common cold should also avoid such food.

6. Sheep

An animal belonging to the bovida family, with different species such as goat, sheep, wild goat, Mongolian gazelle, etc.

Nature and flavour: Mutton, sweet and hot; and bile, bitter and cold.

Constituents: Mutton is rich in protein, fat, inorganic salt and vitamins. Its liver is rich in vitamin A.

Actions: Mutton is nourishing and warming and is beneficial to weakness and helpful to digestion; and its liver, good for eyesight. When stewed with angelica sinensis, it is especially good for postpartum mothers. Its horn in capable of eliminating evil wind and is an antipyretic.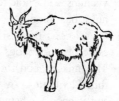

Recipe examples: For the infirm, puerperant. Mutton is a very old traditional blood tonic in traditional Chinese medicine. As early as nearly 2,000 years ago, Chinese physicians formulated a "Mutton Decoction with Radix Angelica Sinensis" for the puerperant in a deficient cold state and susceptible to cold pathogen invasion. Mutton is not only nourishing, but also warm. Use 30 g Radix Angelica Sinensis, 60 g fresh ginger, 500 g mutton. Cut the meat into cubes and cook with other ingredients until well done, then add Chinese onion, salt and flavourings. Consume in 1-2 meals.

(2) For postpartum deficiency with cold limbs, sweating and short breath. Use 500 g mutton cut into larger cubes. Dip in boiling water for 1 minute. Skim off anything floating on the surface. Cut 150 g Chinese yam in rectangular shape and boil with the mutton. Add Chinese onion white, ginger, peppermint, and millet wine. First boil with strong fire and then with slow fire until the mutton is well done. Consume for 2-3 meals.

(3) For anorexia in the elderly. Boil 100 g mutton and skim the floating foamy materials. Cut into small pieces and put in water. Add Chinese onion bulb, ginger and boil until mutton is well done. Pour in 150 g flour, 20 g powdered tangerine peel and stir thoroughly to make paste. Add some salt and monosodium glutamate and serve.

(4) For night blindness. Use 300 g sheep's liver. Cut off the white tissues and slice into thin slices. Boil with 100 g rice to make porridge and serve.

(5) For anemia. Take one femur bone from a sheep and pound to expose its marrow. Boil in water for 1 hour. Add 30 g Chinese dates and 100 g glutinous rice to make porridge. After done, add some brown sugar and serve.

7. Cow

An animal belonging to the bovida family, including buffalo, cow, yak, etc.

Nature and flavour: Beef, sweet and warm; and horn, bitter and cold.

Constituents: Beef is rich in protein of good quality, fat, inorganic salt, vitamins and cholesterol. Milk is sweet and cold, and is a very common nutritional food.

Actions: Beef is beneficial to the whole body, especially to tendons and bones, eliminating edema. The milk is good for the heart and lungs, stopping thirst. Its horn is an antipyretic in epidemic diseases and is good for hemoptysis and epistaxis.

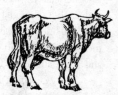

Recipe examples: (1) For the infirm. Slice 100 g beef into thin slices and cook with 50 g rice to make porridge. After done, add some salt and flavourings and eat warm.

(2) For cold spleen and stomach with loss of appetite. Marinade 500-1,000 g beef in the following sauce for 2 hours: Prepare tangerine peel, and Fructus Amomi, each 3 g; fresh ginger 15 g, cinnamon bark 3 g, peppermint 3 g, Chinese onion, salt. Then cook them together in water until well done. Let it cool down and slice to thin pieces, serving as a side dish.

(3) For watery stool due to deficient spleen. Use a complete cow's stomach and 120 g Job's-tears. Simmer with slow fire until beef is well done.

(4) For infirmity and impotence. Use a cow's kidney. Excise all the white tissues. Wrap 50 g rice with gauze. Cook rice and kidney in water to make porridge. When the congee is ready, add salt, fresh ginger and Chinese onion, monosodium glutamate, and consume at one sitting.

8. Dog

An animal belonging to the caninae family.

Nature and flavour: Salt and hot.

Constituents: In addition to protein and fat, as other common animal meat, there are also purine and carnosine, creatine, potassium, sodium and chloride.

Actions: Dog meat is a warm tonic beneficial to the kidney, *qi* and *yang* principle. Hence, it is applied in flatulence of deficient and cold type, edema, malaria of cold nature, the infirm and the elderly.

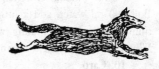

Recipe examples: (1) For kidney deficiency with frequent and urgent urination, emission, cold in the uterus causing sterility. Cut 250 g dog meat into small pieces. Put some oil on pan and heat. Fry 50 g garlic slices. Then take it out and set aside. Pour in the meat, 25 g mushrooms (soaked in water in advance), 50 g bamboo shoot, millet wine, soya bean sauce, sugar, Chinese onion, fresh ginger, sesame oil and 500 ml meat broth. Simmer for 1 hour. Add some peppermint powder and serve.

(2) For edema and ascitis. Cook 500 g dog fat meat with 100 g rice, some salt and fermented soya bean. When well done, comsume with no salt added.

(3) For impotence and cold limbs and lumbago. Simmer 150 g dog meat. Add 12 g cinnamon bark, 12 g tangerine peel, some fresh ginger and salt when well done. Eat the meat and drink the soup at one sitting.

9. Rabbit

An animal belonging to the eporidae family. Its meat, liver and brain are all used for medicinal purposes.

Nature and flavour: Sweet and cool.

Constituents: Rich in protein. Each 100 g meat contains 21.2 g protein, 16 mg, calcium and 2 mg iron.

Actions: Meat is good for general weakness. The brain possesses oxytocic action. The liver improves eyesight, and relieves night blindness and dizziness.

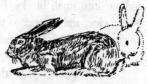

Recipe examples: (1) For infirmity and strengthening the spleen. Prepare 200 g rabbit flesh, 30 g Chinese yam, 15 g fruits of Chinese wolfberry, 15 g dangshen and 30 g Chinese red date. Cook together with slow fire for half an hour and serve.

(2) For thirst of *yin* deficiency type. Prepare a whole rabbit with hair, paws and inner viscera discarded. Cook with Chinese yam to obtain concentrated broth. Drink at any time when thirsty.

(3) For vitamin A deficiency manifesting night blindness or dermatosis. Boil 200 ml water, add a little salt and oil. Place 2 rabbit livers sliced into thin sheets into the boiling water. Pour in a thoroughly stirred hen's egg. When liver well done, consume the whole soup.

10. Carp

A fish belonging to the cyprinidae family, with different colours: yellow, white and red.

Nature and flavour: Sweet and moderate.

Constituents: Containing protein, fat, calcium, phosphorus, vitamins A, B_1, B_2 and C, and nicotinic acid.

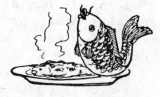

Actions: Nourishing, benefitting digestion and improving milk secretion and diuretic. A sedative for pregnant women and promotes milk secretion.

Recipe examples: (1) For edema due to hepatic or nephritis (nephritic) disorders. Treat a 500 g carp as usual and clean it. Pour in 350 ml vinegar and boil with slow fire until vinegar totally evaporated. Eat the carp, once daily.

(2) For promoting lactation. Treat a carp as usual and clean it. Simmer it in water. When half done, add salt and a little vinegar. Eat the fish and drink the soup.

(3) For short breath and chronic cough. Treat a carp in usual way. Clean and cut into small blocks. Fry in oil to brown. Add soya bean sauce, sugar, millet wine, and simmer to well done. Place in dish and pour marinade made of vinegar, garlic, chives and ginger onto the fish. Serve as a side dish.

11. Cuttlefish (Inkfish)

A fish belonging to the sepiada family. It has a solitary bone in its interior.

Nature and flavour: Salt and slightly warm.

Constituents: Containing protein, with calcium carbonate and mucin in its bone.

Actions: Nourishing. The bone is a hemostat, an astringent and an ideal antacid.

Recipe examples: (1) For nourishing puerperant and promoting milk secretion. Treat an inkfish by discarding its external membrane and inner bone. Also treat a hen as usual. Simmer both in water and add some salt, fresh ginger and other flavourings. Consume in 2-3 meals.

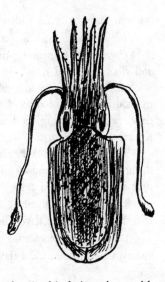

(2) For amenorrhea. Cook a treated inkfish with 10 pieces of peach nut. Drink the soup and eat the inkfish.

(3) For epigastric pain due to peptic ulcer. Clinical reports reveal that the bone of inkfish, when applied with fritillary bulb in a ratio of 85:15 in powder form, yields very satisfactory results in peptic ulcer. The dosage is 2-5 g, three times a day before each meal.

12. Snakehead fish

A fish belonging to the mura enesocidae family, black in colour with small scales.

Nature and flavour: Sweet and cold.

Constituents: Containing protein, fat, calcium, phosphorus, and vitamins A and B.

Actions: Benefitting spleen and stomach. Diuretic and eliminating edema. Hence, it is usually applied in edema, either due to cardiac or kidney diseases.

Recipe example: For edema due to either heart or kidney diseases. Treat a snake head fish with its scales, fins and inner viscera excluded. Simmer in water with 15 g Job's-tears until both are well done. Consume both the soup and fish at one sitting.

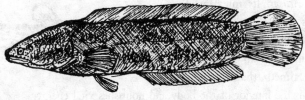

13. Finless eel

A fish belonging to the branchio sauridae family, yellow in colour, without scales, covered with mucous.

Nature and flavour: Sweet, hot.

Constituents: Containing protein, fat, inorganic salt, essential amino acids, and vitamins A and B.

Actions: Beneficial to vital energy, nourishing the blood and general deficiency strenthening the bone and tendon.

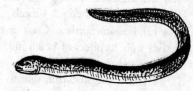

Recipe examples: (1) For strengthening bones and tendons. Treat a finless eel as usual and cut it into segments 3 cm long. Add 15 g dangshen, 9 g Radix Angelica Sinensis, 15 g ox's tendon. Simmer all ingredients until well done. Add some flavourings, salt and serve at one sitting.

(2) For prolapse of anus or uterus. Treat an eel as usual and simmer in 200 ml water. Add salt and flavourings. After done, consume all the soup and eel.

(3) For chronic diarrhoea. Treat the eel as usual and bake on a new tile to dry and then grind with brown sugar into powder. Swallow 5-10 g, twice a day.

(4) For facial paralysis with wry mouth. Kill an eel and obtain some blood. Rub it on the affected side of the face.

14. Loach

A fish belonging to the cobitidae family.

Nature and flavour: Sweet and moderate.

Constituents: Containing rich protein, low fat, vitamins A, B and B_2, iron, and calcium.

Actions: Its mucilaginous secretion is bacterial inhibiting and anti-inflammatory. In TCM, it is claimed that loach

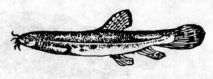

warms the interior of the body and nourishes vital energy.

Recipe examples: (1) For chronic hepatitis. Treat several loaches as usual by thorough cleaning. Place in a pot and add water, 100 g bean curd, flavouring, salt and simmer it. Consume the whole thing, once daily for a week. If a second course is needed, it should be started after 2 days, interval.

(2) For night sweating. Clean 60 g loach and cook it. Make porridge with rice and the loach. Consume it at one sitting.

(3) For thirst due to diabetes. Dry some loaches in the shadow and bake dry. Grind into powder. Grind equal amount of dry lotus leaves into powder and mix together. Use 6 g, 3 times a day.

15. Tortoise

An animal belonging to the testudinidae family. Its abdominal plate is most commonly used for medicinal purposes.

Nature and flavour: Sweet and moderate.

Constituents: Containing protein, fat, vitamins B_1 and B_2.

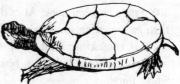

Actions: Nourishing *yin* and blood. It is used in anemia infirmity, tuberculosis with chronic coughing, chronic malaria and bloody stool.

Recipe examples: (1) For *yin* deficiency with insomnia, palpitation. Prepare 250 g turtle meat, 50 g lily, 10 red dates. Simmer the ingredients until the meat is well done. Drink the soup and eat the meat.

(2) For lumbago due to kidney deficiency. Prepare 250 g turtle meat, 100 g walnut, with 9 g cinnamon twigs and simmer them together. Serve after well done.

(3) For prolapse of uterus, stomach or anus. Simmer 250 g turtle meat with 15 g fruit of citron together, and serve.

16. Soft-shelled turtle

An animal belonging to the trionychidae family. The whole body, especially its abdominal plate, is used for medicinal purposes.

Nature and flavour: Salty and moderate.

Constituents: Containing gelatinous protein, fat, kerain, sugar, inorganic salt, iodine, calcium and vitamins A, B, B_2 and D.

Actions: Good for tuberculous fever, eliminating lumps in abdomen in chronic malaria. Its blood nourishes the *yin*-

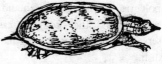

167

principle (vital essence of the body) and reduces fever.

Recipe examples: (1) For *yin* deficiency, manifesting dizziness vertigo, emission, lumbago. Let out the blood of a soft-shelled turtle from dorsal side of its neck. Then, excise at its abdomen to expose the internal viscera which are discarded. The head is also eliminated. Dip in boiling water so as to peel out the black skin on its back and white skin on its abdominal wall. Cut into small cubes. Simmer the turtle flesh in water, and add 30 g Fructus Amomi, 30 g Chinese yam, processed Radix Rehmanniae, some ginger and Chinese onion segments. Before done, discard the onion and ginger slices, add monosodium glutamate. Add peppermint and serve.

(2) For prolapse of anus. Treat a soft-shelled turtle as usual. Simmer with 500 g pig's large intestine. After done, add salt and other flavourings. Eat the flesh and intestine and drink the broth.

(3) For ascitis. Treat a soft-shelled turtle as above. Discard the viscera and head. Simmer with 12 g betel nut and some garlic clove. Consume the whole thing.

Remarks: It is interesting to note that during the last couple of years, it was disclosed that Chinese women long-distance runners who broke the world records have used soft-shelled turtles as one of their important tonics. This has been attributed as one reason for their remarkable records.

17. Freshwater clam

A shellfish belonging to the anodontae family.

Nature and flavour: Salty and cold.

Constituents: Protein, fat, sugar, calcium, vitamins A, B_1 and B_2. Its shell and pearl contain large amounts of calcium carbonate and magnesium carbonate.

Actions: Stopping thirst, eliminating fever and detoxifying. The nacre is used as a remedy for dizziness and excess of liver function.

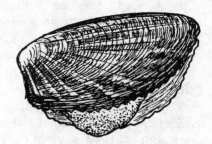

Recipe examples: (1) For thirst and polyuria. Simmer clam flesh and consume it and the broth. It can be served twice daily or as a regular side dish.

(2) For tuberculosis. Prepare 100 g clam flesh, 50 g Chinese chives (hotbed ones). Stir-fry both in oil and serve as a side dish. It can be used as a regular dish.

(3) For *yin* deficiency with dry cough, sore throat, hot palms and soles and night sweats. Boil 100 g clam flesh, 30 g lily, 50 g Chinese yam. After done, add monosodium glutamate and serve.

(4) For beauty purposes. Pearl powder is commonly used as cosmetic for external use. In the Qing imperial palace, pearl powder was used by Empress Dowager Cixi as an important cosmetic.

18. River snail

A shellfish belonging to the paludinae family.

Nature and flavour: Sweet and cold.

Constituents: Containing protein, inorganic salt, vitamins A, B_1, B_2 and D.

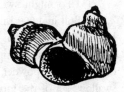

Actions: River snail is beneficial to expel excess and evil fluid in the body and is used as a diuretic. Since it is cold in nature, it relieves summer heat and fever. It is often applied in icteric diseases, edema, thirst, hemorrhoids, bloody stool, red eyes and topically applied for boils and carbuncles.

Recipe examples: (1) For jaundice and dysuria. Use 10-20 large river snails, use clean fresh water to eliminate the mud. Take out the flesh and mix with some millet wine. Boil in 150 ml water, serve once daily.

(2) For the tipsy. Simmer 20 river snails, treated as above. Add some Chinese onion and fermented soya beans. Boil for 15 minutes and drink the soup.

(3) For dysentery. Dry the flesh from river snail under the sun. Bake it to brown, decoct, and serve 9 g, three times daily.

19. Oyster

A shellfish belonging to the ostreidae family. Both the shell and the flesh are used for medicinal purposes.

Nature and flavour: Salty and slightly cold.

Constituents: The flesh contains sugar, lipoid, vitamins, and fucose; and its shell, calcium carbonate, magnesium, aluminium and ferrous oxide.

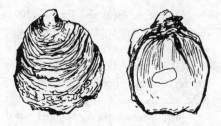

Actions: An excellent nutrient for deficiency of vital essence. Its shell is a sedative and antacid.

Recipe examples: (1) For general weakness and infirmity. Use 200 g oyster flesh, to which 50 g corn starch (or sweet potato starch) is added. Add some fresh water to form a paste. Add some little pieces of fresh garlic with green leaves (garlic clove may be used when fresh ones not available). Fry in oil until brown. Add flavouring sauce and serve. This may be served once daily.

(2) For nervousness. 100 g oyster flesh treated as above. Boil oyster paste in water. Add salt and ginger and serve.

(3) For night sweat, insomnia. Wrap 15 g powdered oyster shell with gauze. Boil in 1,000 ml water under slow fire until only 400-500 ml water is left. Use the decoction as one would tea.

(4) For loss of appetite, ejaculation and night sweat. Mix equal amount of oyster shell powder and wheat bran. Cook 200 g pork. With its broth, swallow 3 g of the mixed powder.

20. Jellyfish

Belonging to the rhopilemada family.

Nature and flavour: Salty and moderate.

Constituents: Containing protein, fat, sugar, inorganic salt and vitamins B_1 and B_2 and nicotinc acid.

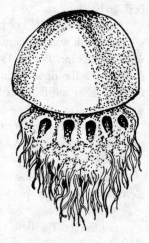

Actions: In animal experiments, it has been shown to lower blood pressure. In TCM, it is claimed that it softens hard masses, eliminates sputum and cures wind and heat in children.

Recipe examples: (1) For hypertension with constipation. Decoct 50 g jellyfish, 4 pieces of water chestnut together for 20 minutes. Consume the whole decoction.

(2) For bronchitis with yellow thick phlegm and coughing. Simmer 100 g jellyfish, 50 g water chestnut. Discard the jellyfish and drink the solution with the water chestnut.

(3) For promoting lactation. Rinse 200 g lettuce and cut into chips. Cut 50 g jellyfish into filaments. Dip both into boiling water for 2 minutes. Place in a dish and add monosodium glutamate, soyabean sauce, sesame oil, vinegar and fresh ginger filaments. Mix thoroughly and serve as a side dish. This can be used twice a day for several days.

E. Processed Foods and Flavourings

1. Salt

There are different kinds of salt produced from sea, well and lake water, as well as rock salt.

Nature and flavour: Salty and cold.

Constituents: Mainly sodium chloride. There are more impurities in sea water salt, such as considerable amount of iodine, potassium chloride, magnesium sulphate, magnesium chloride, calcium sulphate, etc.

Actions: It possesses the actions of clearing evil heat and cooling down evil heat in the blood. It is also an antidote and a very common flavouring. It is essential to body health. No one can lead a normal life without taking salt regularly. It is extensively applied for chest distension, sore throat and

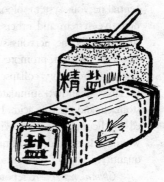

bleeding from the gum. It also stimulates one's appetite and arouses delicious taste.

Recipe examples: (1) For sore throat and habitual constipation. Dissolve 1-2 g salt in 200 ml warm boiled water. Drink in early morning on empty stomach.

(2) For sunstroke with thirst and profuse sweating. Use appropriate amount of salt and sugar and dissolve in warmed boiling water. Drink as one would tea.

(3) For poor milk secretion in puerperant. Fry 50 g black sesame and 25 g salt until sesame is done. Grind into powder form and eat as one likes or with other foods.

(4) For hiccups as a result of immoderate meal. Lick a little salt and place it on surface of tongue. As it dissolves, swallow it bit by bit.

2. Alcoholic drinks

There are a great variety of alchoholic drinks used, including Chinese white liquor, wine, rice or millet wine, etc.

Nature and flavour: Sweet, pungent, warm or hot.

Constituents: Its main contents are ethyl alcohol and water. Different kinds of alcoholic drinks contain various concentrations of ethyl alcohol, ranging from 10-70 percent, and other ingredients, including organic acids such as formic acid, ethyl actate, glycerol, tartaric acid, malic acid, glucose and many others.

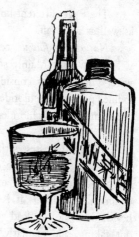

Actions: Alcoholic drinks yield actions on central nervous system, blood circulatory system, digestive system and others. It first excites and then inhibits the nervous system; dilates blood vessels in the skin, promotes circulation and may result in circulatory collapse when administered in large quantity; stimulates secretion of the stomach and gastric acid. Hence, it is indicated in rheumatism, cold evils in the abdomen, wounds. It should be administered in suitable quantity.

Clinical reports: A report mentioned that 14 cases of simple postpartum diarrhoea were treated by boiling 250 ml millet wine to which 125 g brown sugar was added. Continue to boil for 2-3 minutes. Consume it in a draught after cooling down. Ten cases were cured; some within 3 days. Aside from mild vertigo, no side effects were observed.

Recipe examples: (1) Coughing due to cold sputum. Soak pig fat, sesamic oil, bee honey and powdered tea, each 125 g, in liquor. Boil and let cool down.

(2) For itching rash in woman. Mix some bee honey with millet wine

and drink it.

(3) For postpartum simple diarrhoea. Boil 250 g millet wine and add some brown sugar. Boil for another 2-3 minutes. Drink in a draught or in 2 doses.

(4) For rheumatism or pain over the whole body. Fry 500 g black soya beans until it cracks. Soak in 100 ml millet wine in an earthenware pot. Let it cool down and drink.

Remarks: Long term consumption of liquor is harmful to your body's health, especially in excessive amounts. Liquor is called "poisonous" in traditional Chinese medicine.

3. Vinegar

Commonly produced by fermentation of grains, hence the name rice vinegar. There are different kinds of vinegar due to the different processing methods and original materials used.

Nature and flavour: Sour and warm.

Constituents: It mainly contains acetic acid, acetoin, acetaldehyde, formaldehyde, acetal, oxalic acid, lactic acid, acetones and some sugars.

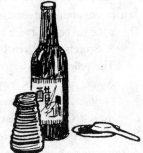

Actions: It possesses the actions of dissipating blood stasis, hemostatic, anditoxic and flavouring. Hence, it is applied in postpartum collapse, lumps, jaundice, and hemoptysis. It also stimulates appetite. It yields refreshing action on the brain with vapor inhalation.

Recipe examples: (1) For ascaris in the biliary ducts. To 30-60 ml vinegar, add warmed boiled water, and drink in a draught.

(2) For acute or chronic hepatitis. Prepare 500 g fresh pig's ribs and place into 1,000 ml vinegar with 125 g brown or white sugar. Boil the vinegar for 30 minutes. Obtain the solution. For adults, 30-40 ml and 10-15 ml for children 5-10 years of age, 3 times daily after meals for 1 month as a therapeutic course. Three courses may be administered.

(3) For jaundice. Use 100 ml vinegar in which 30 g root of membranous milk vetch, 6 g cinnamon twigs and 20 g root of herbaceous peony are added. Pour in some water and boil it. Drink the decoction, once a day for 7 days.

4. Processed soybean

Made by the fermentation of boiled black beans.

Nature and flavour: Bitter and cold.

Constituents: Protein and vitamins B_1 and B_2.

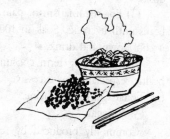

Actions: Antipyretic, and diaphoretic to relieve the exterior syndrome. Detoxifying and promoting eruption of rash in measles.

Recipe examples: (1) For seasonal febrile disease with high fever and skin rash. Use 15 g glutinous rehmannia, 20 g fermented soyabean with 30 g pig's fat. Boil in 150 ml water until 50 ml is left, and drink at a draught.

(2) For dysentery. Use 50 g fermented soyabean and a handful of Alli Macrostem's bulb cut into small pieces. Boil in 150 ml water for 20 minutes. Drink the decoction twice a day.

5. Scorched rice crust

The yellow crust formed at the bottom of the pan when cooking rice.

Nature and flavour: Sweet, moderate, and slightly warm.

Constituents: Mainly starch.

Actions: Good for digestion, and promoting the secretion of digestive fluids. Dyspepsia due to irregular eating and drinking, loss of appetite, chronic gastroenteritis are the most common indications.

Recipe examples: (1) For dyspepsia. Prepare 100 g rice crust, 12 g inner lining membrane of chicken gizzard, 15 g Job's-tears. Boil the last two ingredients in 150 ml water for 20 minutes. Then, add the crust into the boiling solution, and boil for another 2 minutes. Discard the gizzard and consume the other ingredients with the solution. This might be served once daily for a week.

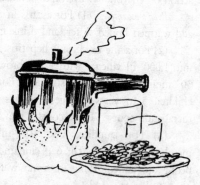

(2) For general weakness of the body. Prepare 100 g rice crust, 30 g shrimp, 50 g lean pork, a tomato, 15 g mushrooms, 5 g water-soaked dry black fungus and other flavourings. Treat and clean all the ingredients in the usual way. Boil 200 ml water to which some corn (or sweet potato) starch dissolved in half cupful of water is added. Stir at the same time when adding the wet corn starch so as to make a thick soup. Add the lean sliced pork, shrimp mushrooms and sliced tomatoes into the soup. Boil for another 2 minutes. Then add a few Chinese onions, salt, monosodium glutamate and fresh ginger filaments. A thick soup is thus formed. Place the crust in a large bowl. Pour the thick soup onto the crust and serve.

Remarks: Over-scorched rice crust (or even charcoal form) is not applicable and should be avoided because there are carcinogenic substances thus produced.

6. Sugar

Made from sugar cane or beets. There are different kinds of sugar, including brown, white and rock.

Nature and flavour: Brown sugar, sweet and warm; and rock sugar, sweet and moderate.

Constituents: Mainly sucrose. There is also chlorophyll, xanthophyll, carrotene and inorganic salt in brown sugar.

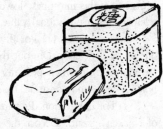

Actions: Benefitting the spleen, vital energy circulation and good for digestion. In addition, it relieves pain, promotes blood circulation and removes stagnation.

Recipe examples: (1) For prevention of sunstroke. Boil 50 g green beans in water until well done. Add a little white sugar and serve.

(2) For diarrhoea due to evil cold. Prepare 50 ml millet wine and 10 g brown sugar. Boil together until the brown sugar dissolves. Drink at a draught.

(3) For pharyngitis, laryngitis and coughing due to evil heat. Peel a piece of flesh from a whole orange. Put 15 g rock sugar into the interior of the orange. Replace the peel in the original site and fix it with a toothpick. Steam the orange in a bowl and consume.

7. Honey

Made by honey bees, which are domesticated. Wild bee honey is also occasionally used.

Nature and flavour: Sweet and moderate.

Constituents: The contents are very complicated. Apart from glucose, fructose and mallose, there is dextrin, protein, iron, calcium, phosphorus, potassium, manganese, sodium, copper, wax, pigments, natural flavouring, malic acid, lactic acid, formic acid, oxidase, transformase and vitamins A, B_1, B_2, B_6, D, E and K.

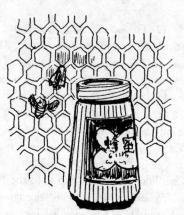

Actions: Nourishing the vital energy, benefitting digestion, and regulating the spleen-stomach function. Easing all the internal viscerae, detoxification. Moistening the intestines, lowering blood pressure and preventing arteriosclerosis. High nutritional value.

Recipe examples: (1) For dry coughing, dry mouth, hot soles and palms due to *yin* deficiency. Dig out the nucleus of a large pear (may be substituted by white turnip when pear not available). Fill in the cavity with 30 g bee honey. Steam and consume, twice daily for several days.

(2) For indigestion. Prepare 30 g Chinese yam and 9 g inner membrane of chicken gizzard. Decoct the two ingredients for 20 minutes. Obtain the solution to which 15 g honey is added and serve, once daily.

(3) For constipation. Prepare 20 g black sesame and 30 g bee honey. Fry the sesame and then pound it as paste. Swallow the paste and honey with warmed boiled water twice daily.

(4) For peptic ulcer. Decoct 9 g licorice, 6 g tangerine peel in 150 ml water for 15 minutes. Discard the residue and pour into 50 g honey and drink, 3 times daily. This can be applied for a considerably long period.

(5) For asthmatic cough. Prepare 30 g fresh ginger juice, 30 g almond. Use some lard to boil the almond. Pound the almond as paste to which ginger juice, honey and sugar, each 15 g, are added. Prepare as bolus in the size of an apricot stone. Eat 6-7 times daily.

Appendix 1

Manifestations of Cold, Heat, Deficiency and Excesses in Traditional Chinese Medicine

Manifestations

High fever, thirst, low voice, constipation, yellow coating on the tongue, red tongue, swift and forceful pulse, sore throat, deep coloured urine, and flushed face.   Heat due to excess

Heat syndrome

Low fever, not thirst, afternoon fever, fatigue, emaciation, scarlet tongue without coating, minute and rapid pulse, and general weakness.   Heat due to deficiency

Cold extremities, abdominal pains, constipation, sunken and string like pulse, and white coating on the tongue.   Cold due to excess

Cold syndrome

Loss of appetite, profuse saliva secretion, shortness of breath, diarrhoea with undigested food, pale tongue with white coating, minute and weak pulse.   Cold due to deficiency

Appendix 2

Manifestations of Excess and Deficiency in Blood and Vital Energy (*Qi*)

Excess syndrome	*Deficiency syndrome*	
Pallor, lassitude, fatigue and weakness, shortness of breath when moving, dizziness, sweating, and diarrhoea. Sometimes prolapses of anus or uterus.	Accumulation and obstruction of phlegm, chest and abdominal distention, vomiting with gastric acid, constipation (clinically termed stagnation of vital energy, and excess syndrome of viscerae)	Vital energy (*qi, yang*)
Paleness in face, lips, tongue and nails, numbness and spasm of extemities, nausea, dizziness, palpitation, restlessness, insomnia, night sweating, afternoon fever, hotness in palms and soles.	Abdominal pains during menstruation or postpartum period, tenderness in abdomen. Local blood stagnation and pain after fall (clinically termed blood stagnation)	Blood (*yin*)

Note: Those patients with *qi* or *yang* deficiency should take diets of moderate and warm nature; those with blood or *yin* deficiency, sweet diets of cold, and cool nature.

Appendix 3

Nature of Everyday Food
(in alphabetical order)

Moderate (or neutral)

Bean
  black bean
  hyacinth bean
  soya bean
  string bean
Bottle-gourd
Carambola
Carp
Carrot
Cauliflower
Cherry
Chicken (flesh)
Chrysanthemum
Cowpea
Date
Egg
Fruit
  Chinese wolfberry fruit
  gorgon fruit
  white mulberry fruit
Gingko
Guava
Honey
Inkfish
Lily
Loach

Pea
Peach
Peanut
Pigeon
Plum, black
Pomelo
Pork
Porridge, rice
Potato, sweet
Pumpkin
Rabbit
Raisin
Rice
Rock-sugar
Sauce, soybean
Seasame
Seed
  lotus seed
  sunflower seed
  watermelon seed
Spinach
Sprout
  bean sprout (soyabean, green bean)
  wheat sprout
Taro
Tea

Loquat
Maize
Milk

Tomato
Tortoise
Turtle, soft-shell
Water chestnut
Wheat, old
Yam, Chinese

Cold

Banana
Bean, mung
Cabbage
Clams
Cogongrass root
Crab
Cucumber
Curd, soya bean
Frog
Fungus, dry black

Hawthorn
Kelp
Milk, soya bean
Pear
Peppermint
Shrimp
Snail (fresh water)
Snake
Soda water (7-Up)

Cool

Almond
Apple
Bamboo shoot
Barley
Beer
Cabbage
Celery
Cocacola
Coconut
Corn
Curd, dried-bean
Duck
Eel
Egg, preserved duck's
    salted duck's

Millet
Noodle (flour)
Orange
Oyster
Persimmon
Pineapple
Salt
Sea cucumber
Seaweed
Sorghum, husked
Tremella
Watermelon
Wax-gourd

Eggplant
Fish (including jellyfish)
Grape
Ice cream
Job's tear

Hot

Black-bone chicken
Butter
Chilli
Chocolate
Clove
Coffee
Curry
Dog's meat
Lamb
Lard
Lichee

Liquor
Longan
Mango
Mustard
Noodle (fried)
Onion
Peanut (fried)
Pepper (white and black)
Prickly ash (Chinese)
Whisky

Warm

Abalone
Aniseed
Beef
Brown sugar
Cheese
Chestnut
Chive
Chocolate milk
Coriander
Crust rice
Flour
Garlic
Ginger
Goose
Ham

Leek
Pomegranate
Potato
Rabbit
Sausage
Shallot
Tangerine
Turkey
Walnut
Wheat (fresh)
Wine (grape, millet and rice)

图书在版编目 (CIP) 数据

中医饮食疗法：英文/蔡景峰著. —修订版.

北京：外文出版社，1996

ISBN 7－119－01885－X

Ⅰ.中… Ⅱ.蔡… Ⅲ.食物疗法—英文 Ⅳ.R247.1

中国版本图书馆 CIP 数据核字 (96) 第 06507 号

中医饮食疗法

蔡景峰　著

*

ⓒ外文出版社

外文出版社出版

（中国北京百万庄大街 24 号）

邮政编码 100037

北京外文印刷厂印刷

中国国际图书贸易总公司发行

（中国北京车公庄西路 35 号）

北京邮政信箱第 399 号　邮政编码 100044

1988 年（34 开）第 1 版

1996 年（大 32 开）第 2 版

（英）

ISBN 7－119－01885－X /R·136（外）

01700

14－E－2144P